BADDITIVES!

BADDITIVES!

The 13 Most Harmful Food Additives in Your Diet—and How to Avoid Them

Linda Bonvie and Bill Bonvie

Foreword by
James S. Turner

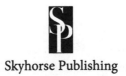

Skyhorse Publishing

Skyhorse Publishing books may be purchased in bulk at special discounts for sales promotion, corporate gifts, fund-raising, or educational purposes. Special editions can also be created to specifications. For details, contact the Special Sales Department, Skyhorse Publishing, 307 West 36th Street, 11th Floor, New York, NY 10018 or info@skyhorsepublishing.com.

Skyhorse® and Skyhorse Publishing® are registered trademarks of Skyhorse Publishing, Inc.®, a Delaware corporation.

Visit our website at www.skyhorsepublishing.com.

10 9 8 7 6 5 4 3 2 1

Library of Congress Cataloging-in-Publication Data is available on file.

Cover design by Jane Sheppard
Cover photo credit: iStock

Print ISBN: 978-1-63450-428-7
Ebook ISBN: 978-1-5107-0034-5

Printed in the United States of America

TABLE OF CONTENTS

FOREWORD

Journalists Linda and Bill Bonvie have been on the food beat for a number of years—most recently as the writers of twice-weekly articles for Citizens for Health's blog *Food Identity Theft* from 2010 to 2015.

Their articles laid out in detail the debasing of the American food supply, for example, by manufacturers using industrial sweeteners such as high fructose corn syrup (HFCS), "flavor enhancers" like monosodium glutamate, and other brain-damaging excitotoxins and artery-clogging trans fats, all of which have been directly linked to the unprecedented health problems that now plague our society.

The articles formed the basis for *Badditives! The 13 Most Harmful Food Additives in Your Diet—and How to Avoid Them*, which zeroes in on the worst of the unnatural substances currently found in processed foods, how they got there, and the ways in which they impact our health (beginning with the first of the alphabetically ordered chapters, which reveals links between aluminum and Alzheimer's disease).

Such ingredients give mechanized foods false color, taste, texture, and stability. Without them most of such processed products would taste bland and appear pale, limp, and inert. Various performance-enhancing chemicals, however, can turn these pasty, unappealing, nutrition-deficient discharges from processing machines into the brightly colored, happy-tasting, feel-good stuff we put into our mouths and call food. They carry real risks, as do other substances covered in the following pages, such as GMOs and fluoride, that adulterate our food for even more devious reasons. Along with chronicling how these badditives came to be accepted by federal regulators, the authors advise you on how to banish them from your diet and thus avoid the pitfalls of the easy, lazy, incurious shopping habits that Big Food encourages.

The industrialization of food has resulted in poor-quality and inherently dangerous products, whose seemingly low prices ultimately translate into much higher healthcare costs. The steady rise of the sale of high fructose corn syrup, for instance, tracks almost exactly the rise of obesity and diabetes in America. In the year following the FDA's politically-engineered approval of the sweetener aspartame (marketed as Equal and NutraSweet), the number of deadly brain tumors rose by 10 percent, reflecting what happened in laboratories when it was fed to test animals. Such have been the results of casual consumption of these and other badditives covered in this book.

"The decline of true taste for food is the beginning of a decline in a national culture as a whole. When people have lost their authentic personal taste, they lose their personality and become the instruments of other people's wills." So said the poet Robert Graves. What this book reveals are the ways in which our declining "true taste for food" have gradually eroded our own will and substituted in its place that of corporate interests. Each of the chapters tells a story of how the goals of making money—and, in some cases, protecting the credibility of regulatory agencies and even shielding a government program from liability—have superseded the original purpose of providing people with nutritious food.

Since 1970, the year I finished my first book, *The Chemical Feast: The Nader Report on Food Protection at the FDA*, the American eating experience has become both better and worse.

On one hand, food manufacturers annually spend billions lobbying for labeling, quality, and safety loopholes in laws and regulations, inundating consumers with false and misleading advertising, and manipulating science to support their profiteering practices. Some of their best and brightest employees work sixty-hour weeks to pass off prettified sludge as healthy food, industrial ooze as sugar, ammonia-treated beef scraps as meat, and adulterated, empty-calorie snacks as sources of nutrition. Food and chemical companies also block consumers from knowing about the presence in their food of genetically modified organisms (GMOs) and cancer-causing bovine growth hormone (rBGH), as well as industrial waste added to water and disguised as a beneficial substance (fluoride). They block, distort, ridicule, and vilify all research that raises even the slightest question about these practices and their lucrative and fanciful food quality and safety claims.

On the other hand, since 1970, a number of reforms and developments have increased our ability to find safer and more nutritious foods. Among them were the Nutrition Labeling and Education Act (NLEA), which abolished the FDA's ban on health claims for food, providing a somewhat better path to quality food advertising, and the Organic Food Production Act, which established rules for a parallel quality food system that has since established a substantial presence in conventional food outlets. The Dietary Supplement Health and Education Act (DSHEA) has also recognized and empowered a supplement market for nutrition lost during manufacturing, and the demand for locally grown food has surged.

The outlines of the struggle to preserve real food in the face of industrialized methods of production will soon become apparent to the reader of this book. The first great food revolution came with the invention of agriculture, followed many centuries later by the Industrial Revolution's attempts to tame and harness agricultural production. Currently, we find ourselves in the midst of what the late futurist Alvin Toffler called the "Third Wave information revolution." The challenge faced by today's consumers is to use the information that revolution has made available to them in choosing the best and healthiest products on the market and rejecting those that have resulted in obesity, illness, and premature death.

However, make no mistake—the food additive/chemical/pharmaceutical industries are working tirelessly on a daily basis to block every effort to help consumers make the wisest choices for their families and their communities. *Badditives!* can be a powerful tool in your own struggle to escape being "the instruments of other people's wills." Read it before your next trip the supermarket—and use it to bolster your power to achieve personal freedom and health.

James S. Turner, Esq.
Chair, Citizens for Health
Washington, DC
July 4, 2016

INTRODUCTION

WHAT THEY'RE NOT TELLING US

It's no secret that eating can be a risky proposition these days.

News reports of periodic outbreaks of incapacitating and sometimes life-threatening ailments caused by pathogens like *Salmonella* and *E. coli*, and the resulting massive products recalls, have become almost routine.

Most often, these involve things like meat and chicken, although no food is immune. Of course, the mainstream media have no hesitation about bringing such threats to our health and safety to our attention as soon as they're made aware of them. That is, after all, part of their job—keeping us informed. And when federal regulators are found to be at fault—for instance, by delaying action in regard to recalls, as the Food and Drug Administration was found to have done in June 2016, shortly before work on this book was completed—we can usually rely on journalists who cover them to give us the heads up.

In recent years, we've also been given frequent warnings that many of the processed foods we buy or eat in restaurants are overloaded with things like sugar, salt, and fat. We're told that these foods simply have too many calories and are informed about the well-meaning campaigns to help us cut down on our consumption of such items.

However, this doesn't mean we're getting the whole story where issues of safety and trustworthiness related to our food supply are concerned, or, for that matter, an entirely accurate one. What we aren't being made aware of—at least, by our everyday news sources—is both shocking and scary. So much so, in fact, that it should be setting off alarm bells among medical and health professionals throughout the land.

In essence, what they're not telling us is that a majority of the attractively packaged, nationally advertised, and reassuringly familiar products on supermarket shelves are largely unfit for human consumption. The reason is that many of the additives they contain—those things usually (but not always) listed among their ingredients, if you take the trouble to look—can have some horrific effects on our health. Hence the name, *Badditives.*

If that's the case, you might ask, where's the evidence? Shouldn't people be keeling over dead after ingesting the products in which these substances are found?

Actually, untold numbers of Americans are dying prematurely every day from preventable diseases that have increasingly been linked to these badditives by researchers. The rates of maladies such as diabetes, nonalcoholic fatty liver disease, and Alzheimer's have skyrocketed (as has that of obesity) since a number of the ingredients discussed in this book were introduced into our food supply. That's not to mention various types of cancers and neurological problems like attention deficit hyperactivity disorder or ADHD—a condition that has gone from being relatively rare a half century ago to so common that students are routinely prescribed dangerous drugs to control it.

Don't expect to be hearing about such things on the six o'clock news, however. The rare exception will be when the FDA is forced to acknowledge that something is amiss and takes steps to correct it, as it finally did in announcing that partially hydrogenated oil (PHO) was to be phased out of processed foods, admitting that it is killing an estimated seven thousand people annually. (As of this writing, however, it's still very much there, which is why we've chosen to include it among the badditives in this book.)

So why aren't we hearing about this from the media, which are always looking for a "scoop?" Why isn't the FDA doing more to keep such harmful substances out of the products it's supposed to be monitoring?

The answer to the first question has a lot to do with the dependency major news outlets have developed on Big Food, as well as on the biotech industry—especially Monsanto, whose own unique role in the toxic transformation of our food will be discussed in the chapters on GMOs and rBGH. (In other words, don't deliberately rock the boat or bite the hand that feeds you.) This is in addition to the fact that many reporters frankly don't have a real handle on the issues involved and tend to fall for fallacies such as the currently popular urban myth that people are simply getting way too much sugar from soft drinks, when what these beverages now actually contain is something far more harmful (as do the supposedly healthier "diet" alternatives).

As for the second question, well, that largely involves politics in the form of the often too-cozy relationship that exists between regulators and those they regulate, one example being the so-called "revolving door" that's enabled top-level officials to shuttle back and forth between the FDA and the industries it's charged with keeping in line.

The purpose of *Badditives!* is to acquaint you with what we have come to regard as the "worst of the worst" in terms of food ingredients, how they came to be an accepted part of our diet, the adverse effects they can have on your health and well-being, and how to steer clear of them. In most cases, of course, the best method of avoiding them is, whenever possible, to buy certified organic products, which not only are grown without chemical pesticides and fertilizers, but are free of most of the substances discussed in this book as well. However, even these aren't perfect, as you'll learn in the chapter on carrageenan, a "natural" ingredient that isn't nearly as harmless as it's made out to be.

Many of the concerns you'll find discussed in these pages have been addressed at length in some excellent books, documentary films, and a good deal of scientific and historical information—some of which is cited here and can also be found on the Internet. (Of course, "Internet rumors" and "conspiracy theories" are two of the favorite terms used by industry propagandists in an attempt to dismiss most of the kind of carefully researched information you'll find here and elsewhere, as if conspiracies—defined as schemes devised by two or more people—were nonexistent, and the Internet was nothing more than a source of unsubstantiated hearsay.) Some of the books we would recommend for those of you who would like to learn more about these issues have been used as references and are mentioned in the chapters that follow.

Hopefully, by the time you finish reading about the damage done by the motley gang of "badditives" to which these chapters are dedicated, you'll realize that there's a lot more to worry about in the products you might assume to be safe than merely the amount of sugar (which is actually used much less than it was in years past), sodium (a certain amount of which is actually necessary to keep us alive), and calories they contain. And once you start examining the lists of ingredients on food packages (if you're not already doing so), you'll see just how many of them are out there waiting for you and your family to ingest—often half a dozen or more strong in a single product.

At that point, you'll realize it's well worth the effort to bar them permanently from your home, your life, and your body.

Linda Bonvie and Bill Bonvie
Tuckerton, New Jersey
June, 2016

ALUMINUM

The Metallic Menace
to Your Mentality

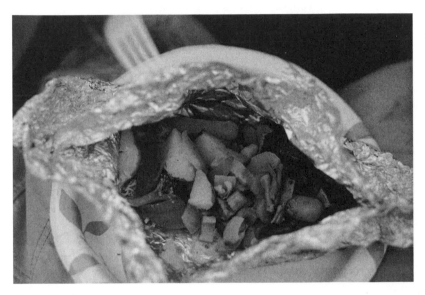

Credit: iStock

"How do we know that Alzheimer's disease is not the manifestation of chronic aluminum toxicity in humans?"
—Professor Christopher Exley, Keele University, UK

Ask anyone over a certain age what they're most afraid of when it comes to their health, and they'll probably tell you it's Alzheimer's. Yet, many of us regularly and casually consume things containing an ingredient that's now being directly linked to that dreaded, mind-robbing disease.

In fact, you're probably doing so yourself and are not even aware of it. Because the ingredient in question—aluminum—can be found in a whole bevy of processed foods, ranging from frozen fish to commercial cake mixes, not to mention various over-the-counter drugs, cosmetics, and grooming products, such as antiperspirants. Its permitted uses in food items include serving as a firming agent, coloring agent, anticaking agent, buffer, neutralizing agent, dough strengthener, emulsifying agent, stabilizer, thickener, leavening agent, curing agent, and texturizer.[1]

Like other substances of questionable safety, this most commonplace of metals came into widespread use in consumer products during the post–World War II period. In various forms, it was officially accorded GRAS (generally recognized as safe) status as a food additive by the FDA back in 1959—meaning that as something in "common use" by then, it required no clinical testing or risk-benefit analysis (which translates to: it must be safe, because people have been using it for a while without any immediately apparent ill effects).

In fact, after President Nixon in 1969 directed the FDA to undertake a systematic safety review of all GRAS substances, a select committee of the Federation of American Societies for Experimental Biology (FASEB) was contracted to do a "re-review" on the status of aluminum. The committee concluded: "There is no evidence in the available literature on . . . acidic sodium aluminum phosphate [and other forms of aluminum] . . . that demonstrates, or suggests reasonable grounds to suspect, a hazard to the public when they are used at levels that are now current or that might reasonably be expected in the future."[2]

Interestingly enough, however, although "noting that care should be taken by patients with kidney disease when consuming food containing high levels of Al (aluminum) salts," the authors of that report "did not mention either dialysis encephalopathy, which has been attributed to aluminum, or *the controversial role of Al in Alzheimer's disease*. Description of these clinical problems began about the same time," notes Robert A. Yokel, a University of Kentucky pharmaceutical sciences professor.[3]

Experts began suspecting aluminum as a possible perpetrator in the proliferation of Alzheimer's cases after residues of the metal began turning up in the brains of some individuals who had succumbed to the disease. The connection, in fact, was considered strong enough that back in 2010, a scientist for Egypt's National Organization for Drug Control and Research, looking into the curative effect of coriander (also known as cilantro) on neurodegenerative disorders and Alzheimer's, reported using an aluminum compound to induce those ailments in the cerebral cortex of male albino rats.[4]

But consumers were constantly reassured that there was never enough "proof" of an aluminum–Alzheimer's association to be concerned about it, especially given that the victims were mostly older people and no direct cause-and-effect association was ever clearly established.

All that changed, however, in 2014, when much stronger evidence of such a link emerged—strong enough to move aluminum from something regarded with mere suspicion into the category of an official "suspect."

Finding the forensic evidence

The breakthrough came when researchers from England's Keele University examined the brain of an industrial worker who had died of early-onset Alzheimer's following eight years of regular occupational exposure to aluminum sulfate dust. Prior to his diagnosis, the man, whose medical history showed no indication of the disease, complained of tiredness, headaches, and mouth ulcers, then began to develop memory problems and depression.

Following his death several years later, a neuropathological examination confirmed an advanced stage of Alzheimer's disease. "There then followed the most comprehensive investigation ever of the aluminium [the British spelling] content of the frontal lobe of a single individual with forty-nine different tissue samples being measured for aluminium,"[5] according to a press release from the university.

The examination found the amount of aluminum in the victim's brain to be at least four times higher than what might be expected for someone his age, noted Christopher Exley, a Keele professor of bioinorganic chemistry who has spent thirty years researching the effects of aluminum, during which he has published more than 150 papers on the subject.[6] "Overall, these results suggest very strongly that occupational exposure . . . contributed significantly to the untimely death of this individual with Alzheimer's disease," Exley declared.[7]

As dramatic as this finding was, however, it's not the only one that has convinced Exley of a direct association between aluminum exposure and Alzheimer's. His conclusions are also based on a decade-long, ongoing examination that he and his colleagues have made of that link in more than a hundred human brains—an investigation that they are currently endeavoring to expand by raising funds to conduct an unprecedented clinical trial in collaboration with the Children's Medical Safety Research Institute (aluminum also being an adjuvant in vaccines given to children).[8] While aluminum, according to Exley, "is rarely acutely toxic in human beings,"[9] there comes a point at which "the accumulation of aluminum in the brain will achieve a toxic threshold" when a specific area will start reacting to its presence, rather than coping with it. And if that part of the brain is already affected by any other ongoing degenerative condition, such as Alzheimer's disease, the aluminum may cause it to become more aggressive, "and perhaps to have an earlier onset."[10] (It isn't just Alzheimer's that Exley believes could be promoted by excessive buildup of aluminum in the brain, but neurodegenerative diseases such as Parkinson's and multiple sclerosis as well.[11])

Of course, the amounts of aluminum you're absorbing into your bloodstream from food, as well as antacids and other sources, aren't apt to be anything like the airborne levels to which that unfortunate British worker was exposed. The evidence of aluminum's complicity in the development of Alzheimer's and other neurodegenerative ailments still isn't rock solid, which is what allows the industry to act as if there isn't any. However, given the discovery by expert investigators that this toxic metal is a likely suspect rather than just a "substance of interest," is it really something you want in things you consume on a daily basis?

Studies of laboratory animals have also indicated that excessive aluminum in the diet of pregnant or nursing mothers can result in "developmental deficits" in the brains of their offspring, including motor reflexes, learning capability, and cognitive behavior. That in itself should be enough cause for any woman who's expecting to be especially vigilant about avoiding products that contain it.[12]

"The presence of aluminum in the human brain," warns Exley, "should be a red flag alerting us all to the potential dangers of the aluminum age" in which "we are all accumulating a known neurotoxin in our brain from our conception to our death."[13] But this is one risk that can be largely averted, simply by taking the time to make sure that the foods, drugs, and cosmetics we buy, and the cookware we use, are free of this metallic menace to our mentality.

And if the risk of Alzheimer's wasn't enough . . .

The brain isn't the only organ that researchers believe is adversely affected by aluminum exposure. According to the summary of a report appearing in the June 2016 issue of the French medical journal *Morphologie*, aluminum ingestion affects "the regulation of the permeability, the microflora and the immune function of (the) intestine," and could be "an environmental risk factor for inflammatory bowel diseases."[14] (What makes this especially perverse is the fact that a number of the antacids now on the market, which are often taken for gastric distress, contain aluminum compounds as either active or inactive ingredients—which is why you should check those labels as well.)

The absorption of aluminum in the bones can also contribute to the development of osteoporosis, especially in people with poor kidney function or whose calcium intake is low, by lowering bone density and increasing the risk of fractures.[15]

Aluminum, in other words, appears from all indications to be really, really bad for the health of your brain, your gut, and your bones—but unlike most of the other badditives in this book, the ways in which you can be exposed to it go well beyond food. You therefore need to not only be diligent about looking for it on the labels of processed food products but also on those of antacids and other drugs (such as buffered aspirin), as well as avoiding the use of aluminum cookware and being very careful about not allowing aluminum foil to be used in cooking or to otherwise come in contact with acidic foods. (That's not to mention tossing any antiperspirants you may have been using, as they are actually required to contain aluminum by definition.)

While eliminating the various ways this toxic metal can enter your system may take a small amount of effort, it's an effort that may be essential to maintaining the health of both your mind and body.

The many things that allow aluminum to accumulate in our daily diet

Is there a connection between the skyrocketing rate of Alzheimer's and the many sources of aluminum to which an average American family may be exposed these days on a daily basis? While that question may not yet have a definitive answer, you don't need one to reduce your own family's risk by eliminating products containing this metal from your diet.

The everyday processed food products alone to which aluminum compounds are still being added, as we discovered on a recent supermarket survey, include these popular items:

- The three biggest brands of cake mixes—Betty Crocker, Pillsbury, and Duncan Hines—all of which have sodium aluminum phosphate listed as an ingredient.
- Kellogg's Eggo Nutri-Grain frozen waffles, including such seemingly "healthy" varieties as blueberry and whole wheat.
- Gorton's Original Batter Fish Tenders and Crispy Battered Fish Fillets, both of which list sodium aluminum phosphate as an ingredient.
- Tastykake Mini Donuts, which also contain sodium aluminum phosphate.

Besides products such as these, if you're doing any baking, you might not realize that at least two brands of supermarket baking powder—Davis and Clabber Girl—will add a smidgen of sodium aluminum phosphate to your homemade cakes and pies (as opposed to such brands as Argo and Rumsford, whose labels note that they're "aluminum-free").

Even if you think a product is aluminum-free, if you haven't bought it in a while, you might want to check the ingredients label. Recently, for instance, we were shocked to find that a brand of Irish soda bread we were accustomed to buying for St. Patrick's Day, thinking it was badditive-free, had added an aluminum compound to its list of ingredients.

That's not to mention the extra amount of aluminum you might be ingesting if you use aluminum foil to wrap meats, fish, and other items during cooking, and from aluminum cookware (which can be replaced with newer ceramic varieties).

Know your badditives—and how to avoid them:

ALUMINUM

- When baking, be sure to only use aluminum-free baking powder (it will usually say so on the label).
- Check ingredient lists and avoid products that contain aluminum compounds.
- If you're buying goodies from a bakery, ask them about the baking powder they use. If they don't know, maybe it's time to shop elsewhere.
- When cooking, don't allow aluminum foil to come in contact with food, especially acidic dishes (such as ones containing tomatoes) or ones cooked at high temperatures. Cleaning up might not be as easy, but in the long run it's worth the effort!
- Check your antacids—certain brands can contain large amounts of aluminum.

ARTIFICIAL COLORS

Agents of Food Fraud That Are Putting Kids on the Road to Ritalin

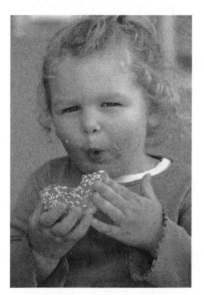

Credit: iStock

"Perhaps, if the FDA had required neurotoxicity testing, especially in young children, before allowing AFCs [artificial food colors] and other additives to be marketed, we would not be having this debate at all. Harvey Wiley, who became the FDA's first commissioner, recruited his legendary 'Poison Squad' volunteers for precisely this purpose. That was in 1902."

—Dr. Bernard Weiss, University of Rochester
Department of Environmental Medicine

Of all the cheap tricks used by food processors to mass-market their commodities while compromising the health of customers, the use of synthetic dyes is the one that really takes the cake when it comes to being flagrantly fake.

While such fakery in the bakery isn't that hard to distinguish, what may be less apparent are many of the packaged products, ranging from cereals to salad dressings, which have had their appearance artificially enhanced through the use of coloring agents made from petroleum derivatives.

Fortunately, a growing number of consumers are no longer falling for this pervasive form of food fraud—especially after being made aware of the behavioral effects it can have on their kids, for whom many of these prettied-up products are intended. A number of major companies, as a result, have begun to respond by simply dispensing with these deceptive dyes and replacing them with more natural substances.

However, that's not to say there aren't plenty of processed foods dressed up in counterfeit colors that still remain on supermarket shelves, many of which are deliberately designed to appeal to preschoolers. That's why we can't afford to let our guard down—and why it's so important to keep up the pressure on the industry to drop the deceptive and damaging disguises they use to lure innocent children and unwary grown-ups.

A history of supposedly "harmless" hues that weren't

The history of artificial colors is one that has long been colored by controversy. Actions to remove them from the food supply are often long overdue. For example:

- Red Dye #2: Considered to be of questionable safety for more than two decades, it was finally banned by the FDA in 1976 after being linked to a statistically significant rise in cancer among laboratory animals.[16]
- Violet #1: Once used not only in cakes, candies, drink powders, and soda, but also in the USDA's purple meat stamp, it

was also banned that same year, fourteen years after a Canadian study found half the rats that ingested it developed cancerous growths.

- Red Dye #3: Despite having been prohibited from cosmetics and externally applied drugs over a quarter century ago, following concerns about its being associated with thyroid cancer in rats, oddly enough it is still allowed to be used in food items, ranging from maraschino cherries and the cherries in fruit cocktail to sausage casings. As nutrition expert and author Dr. Michael Greger observed in 2015, "While FDA scientists and FDA commissioners have recommended that the additive be banned, there has been tremendous pressure to delay the recommendations from being implemented."[17]

It's hardly surprising that so many supposedly "harmless" synthetic hues have been found to be otherwise when you consider their origins and backgrounds. In fact, the passage of the original federal food safety law, the 1906 Pure Food and Drugs Act, was largely designed to curtail the use of hazardous coloring agents to disguise the appearance of various products.

When that law was expanded in 1938, it called for special certification for many of the dyes that were then made from coal tar—a thick, black liquid derived from, well, coal (hardly the sort of ingredient you'd knowingly add to food). While some of those are still in use today, the newer ones are more apt to be petroleum extracts, which may also contain measurable amounts of toxic contaminants, such as lead, mercury, and arsenic.

In spite of those regulatory measures, our processed food products have continued to be colored with synthetic compounds that research is increasingly revealing to be hazardous to our health (and especially that of our children)—badditives that only recently have begun to be replaced with substances more fit for human consumption.

In February of 2015, the country's two best known chocolate candy manufacturers announced they would start phasing unnatural colors out of their products—a long overdue declaration that was an encouraging sign of such synthetic hues fading from the food scene.

First, Nestlé USA announced its commitment to removing FDA-certified colors, like Red #40 and Yellow #5, as well as artificial flavors, from all of its confections—more than 250 products in all, including such standard candy bar brands as Butterfinger, Crunch, Chunky, Raisinets, Goobers, Oh Henry, and Baby Ruth.[18] Not to be outdone, however, Hershey's came out a few days later with its own "clean-label initiative," one that pledged to "transition existing products" to exclude not only artificial colors and flavors, but also high fructose corn syrup and genetically modified ingredients.[19]

A year later, a third big candy maker, Mars, followed suit, announcing that it was removing all artificial colors from "its entire human food portfolio." (While asserting that such coloring agents "pose no known risks to human health or safety," the company said its action was "part of a commitment to meet evolving consumer preferences" for "more natural ingredients" and that it would "work closely with its suppliers to find alternatives that not only meet its strict quality and safety standards, but also maintain the vibrant, fun colors consumers have come to expect" from its brands.)[20]

The country's major candy companies were not the only food enterprises to make such moves away from synthetic hues and flavors. By mid-2015, some of the other best-known names in the industry, including Campbell's Soups, General Mills, and Kraft, were announcing plans to remove either all such artificial ingredients (in the case of Campbell's) or to replace some, like the artificial colors in Trix Cereal and Kraft Macaroni & Cheese, with natural ingredients such as paprika, turmeric, fruit and vegetable juices, and vanilla. A number of fast-food franchises, including Pizza Hut, Taco Bell, Papa John's, and Subway, as well as health-conscious Chipotle, said they were doing likewise.[21]

All this followed an acknowledgment by the FDA that at least 96 percent of children from ages two to five were being exposed to at least four artificial dyes in food products—FD&C Red #40, Yellow #5, Yellow #6, and Blue #1. That announcement came all of six years after a petition was submitted to the agency by the Center for Science in the Public Interest (CSPI), asking that nine such food colorings be banned. The group also demanded the posting of an interim warning label on foods containing them that these dyes "cause hyperactivity and behavioral problems in some children."

"The continued use of these unnecessary artificial dyes is the secret shame of the food industry and the regulators who watch over it," CSPI executive director Michael F. Jacobson said at the time. "The purpose of these chemicals is often to mask the absence of real food, to increase the appeal of a low-nutrition product to children, or both."[22]

Actually, getting that FDA admission was no small accomplishment, given that the agency's initial response to the petition and nearly eight thousand public comments was to convene a Food Advisory Committee, a majority of whose members (57 percent) voted against additional labeling requirements for foods that contain certified color additives. According to an official summary, "The Committee made the determination that relevant scientific data did not support a causal link between consumption of certified color additives in food and hyperactivity and other problematic behaviors in children," and "suggested that additional safety studies, such as developmental neurotoxicity testing of the color additives, be conducted and that a robust intake estimate be calculated."[23]

Red flags in a variety of colors

In the meantime, however, researchers were continuing to confirm "causal links" between the consumption of synthetic food dyes and behavioral problems in kids. The discovery of one such link, in fact, was made by researchers at Yale University's Department of Pediatric Neurology who undertook studies to determine the effects of five common synthetic food dyes on baby rats. However, unlike experiments that have used excessive amounts of the substances in question, these relied on the equivalent of the "real world" exposures our kids have to these dyes. The results were alarming—the rats became hyperactive and showed diminished learning ability (as did those given 6-OHDA, a chemical that reduces dopamine levels in the brain).

According to Dr. Bennett A. Shaywitz, who led the experiment, "whereas animals not exposed to any colors or 6-OHDA took about 9 seconds to escape the maze, it took over twice as long (23 seconds) for the animals exposed to the lower .5 mg/kg artificial color doses to escape the maze (considered a significant difference)."[24]

Nor is this an effect that has been confined to lab rats.

Back in 2007, a randomized, double-blind, placebo-controlled British study, published in the medical journal *The Lancet*, found that artificial food dyes not only increased hyperactivity in children with ADHD, but "in the general population and across the range of severities of hyperactivity."[25] This in turn prompted the American Academy of Pediatricians to acknowledge a link between their consumption and attention deficit hyperactivity disorder (ADHD) and to recommend parents try removing them from the diet of a child who suffers from the condition.[26]

Since then, a number of other studies have substantiated these findings, including a 2013 meta-analysis by a team of international researchers of six nonpharmaceutical ADHD treatment options, which concluded that excluding artificial food colorings from the diet, unlike other options, "produced statistically significant reductions in ADHD symptoms."[27]

The results of yet another meta-analysis—this one done with funding from the International Life Sciences Institute, which is affiliated with the food industry—were used by CSPI at the start of 2016, along with Centers for Disease Control (CDC) data, in "conservatively" estimating that more than half a million children in the US suffer adverse behavioral reactions from food dyes, costing more than $5 billion per year.[28]

In other words, the road to Ritalin could well have been paved with all those FD&Cs you see listed among the ingredients of processed food products.

Not that the link between food dyes, as well as other ingredients, such as aspartame, and behavioral problems in kids hasn't been known and treated for quite some time using the Feingold Program as noted in the study published in *The Lancet* (see box). As is so often the case, however, it took decades for that message to reach the mainstream, during which many thousands of students were prescribed behavioral modification drugs that have started many down the path to addiction. In the meantime, as they have with other additives, European Union regulators beat us to the punch back in 2010 by requiring food products containing these counterfeit colors to carry a warning label stating that consumption "may have an adverse effect on activity and attention in children."[29]

The Feingold Program: A food-based, drug-free approach to ADHD

The connection between certain food additives, such as artificial colors, and problems like hyperactive behavior and lack of concentration was first made by the late Dr. Benjamin Feingold, a California pediatrician and pioneer in the field of allergy and immunology, whose findings were originally presented in 1973 to the American Medical Association.

The Feingold Program he subsequently created has helped scores of kids suffering from ADHD by systematically eliminating certain additives from their diets, all without resorting to the kinds of behavior-modification drugs that are all too often dispensed by school authorities in an attempt to force these kids to pay more attention and stop being disruptive.

Further details about the Feingold program can be found at the website for the Feingold Association of the United States: http://feingold.org/about-the-program/dr-feingold/#

Hyperactivity, however, isn't the only health problem associated with such synthetic dyes. For example:

- Red # 40: A petroleum derivative and the most commonly used artificial color. It has been known to cause a variety of allergic reactions, including hives and swelling of the tongue and face, gastrointestinal distress, and respiratory symptoms, such as chronic sneezing and itching of the nose, eyes, and throat.[30] It also contains a suspected carcinogen.[31] (A natural replacement for Red #40 that is sometimes used, carmine or cochineal extract made from crushed cochineal insects, has also been rejected by many consumers, resulting in an increased demand for a more acceptable, lycopene-based substitute called Tomat-O-Red.[32])
- Yellow #5 (tartrazine): It may cause allergic reactions, especially in those who are hypersensitive to aspirin. It has also been linked to asthma, migraines, fatigue, anxiety, and blurred vision.[33]

- Yellow #6 (sunset yellow): Currently banned in Norway and Finland, it can cause gastrointestinal distress, swelling of the skin, a nettle-type rash, and migraines. It has also reportedly been linked to cancer of the adrenal glands and kidneys.[34]
- Blue #1 (brilliant blue): It may trigger asthma, low blood pressure, hives, and other allergic reactions. It also caused serious complications and death in hospital patients when used in feeding tube solutions several years ago.[35]

Then there's the fact that these dyes characteristically contain trace amounts of toxic substances, such as metals, mercury, and arsenic, which the Feingold Association's Bluebook points out is "reason enough to avoid them."[36]

Given such "toxicological considerations" as carcinogenicity, hypersensitivity reactions, and behavioral effects, CSPI notes in its 2010 report *Food Dyes: A Rainbow of Risks* (available for viewing online) that "food dyes cannot be considered safe." The report therefore urges that the FDA ban these ingredients, "which serve no purpose other than a cosmetic effect," and that the law "be amended to make it no more difficult to ban food colorings than other food additives." In the meantime, it suggests that companies voluntarily replace such dyes with "safer, natural colorings."[37]

To a certain extent, that last recommendation is what's now being implemented. However, it's not happening nearly quickly or comprehensively enough to keep many thousands of America's kids from being subjected to the double whammy of adverse reactions to these particular badditives and the risky drugs given out to treat them.

In other words, it's still up to us to keep these enticing lures—whether in the form of a Red #40-colored "Bright & Lively Strawberry Balsamic Dressing" from Kraft or a box of Keebler's "Rainbow Chips Deluxe" containing no fewer than ten artificial colors—from entering our personal food chain.

Unlike synthetic ones, "true colors" can be a boon to our brains and our bodies

There's a good reason why food manufacturers use colors as a come-on in selling their products—the fact that our palates are probably programmed to respond favorably to the natural ones in Mother Nature's palette.

However, while artificial colors might be harmful to our health, the true hues in food are actually quite beneficial to us in various ways.

Take blueberries, for example. Their blue, purple, and red pigments are actually anthocyanins—powerful antioxidants that can actually do wonders for our brain health and cognitive ability by helping our neurons maintain their lines of communication (just the opposite, in fact, of the effects of consuming artificial colors).

Then there are tomatoes, watermelon, and pink grapefruit, whose reds and pinks are due to the presence of lycopene, considered a potent anticancer agent (and that also goes for processed tomato products like tomato sauce and tomato paste).

Other naturally occurring beneficial hues include the shades of orange and yellow found in veggies such as carrots, pumpkins, and sweet potatoes, which are great sources of beta-carotene, a pigment that not only helps ward off cancer and heart disease but also protects your eyesight and immune system.[38]

Know your badditives and how to avoid them:

ARTIFICIAL COLORS

- Unless you're a diehard consumer of organic processed foods, read the ingredient labels on all processed foods.
- Watch out for what you might be sure are naturally colored foods, such as pickles, cereals, and pizza. Artificial colors can turn up in the strangest places!
- Check ingredient lists on vitamins, particularly those intended for kids, which are likely to contain fake colors.

ASPARTAME

The Dangerous Drug Posing as a "Healthy" Sweetener

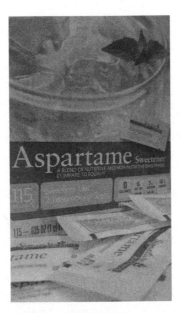

Credit: Linda Bonvie

"As a busy clinician I continue to see the multiple neurological and psychiatric consequences of aspartame use. It can lower seizure threshold and lead to an incorrect diagnosis of epilepsy, with subsequent inappropriate prescription of anticonvulsants. It can mimic or exacerbate symptoms of MS, it can paradoxically produce carbohydrate craving and weight gain."

—Ralph G. Walton, MD, former chairman,
Department of Psychiatry,
Northeastern Ohio Universities College of Medicine

One of the rules governing pharmaceuticals, and their advertising, is that side effects have to be listed. That's the reason drug commercials include all those warnings about possible adverse reactions.

But there's a drug that's been on the market for several decades, one that countless unsuspecting consumers are encouraged to use as a supposedly healthy sweetening agent. It is added to numerous "sugar-free" products, whose only mandatory warning is directed at people who suffer from a relatively rare health problem—a condition called phenylketonuria, or PKU, which affects an estimated 14,500 Americans.[39]

For everybody else, aspartame—a chemical mixture of two amino acids, phenylalanine and aspartate, and methanol (wood alcohol)—is regarded by the US Food and Drug Administration as "safe for the general population." In fact, an agency bulletin describes it as "one of the most exhaustively studied substances in the human food supply, with more than 100 studies supporting its safety."[40]

Unfortunately, that assessment doesn't jibe with thousands of complaints about aspartame's side effects reportedly received by the FDA's Adverse Reactions Monitoring System, as well as many, many more that have been logged by the Aspartame Consumer Safety Network, a Texas-based organization formed in 1987 that no longer actively collects any but the most serious case histories from consumers, according to its founder, Mary Nash Stoddard. "The tens of thousands of documented cases we have in our files convince us we are accurate in our pronouncements that aspartame is harming, and in some cases, killing users around the globe," says Stoddard.[41]

Our attempts to get statistics from current FDA officials were unsuccessful. However, according to Mark Gold, who heads another watchdog group called the Aspartame Toxicity Information Center in Concord, New Hampshire, approximately seven thousand consumers had directly notified the FDA of around ten thousand adverse reactions to the product by 1995, when the agency supposedly stopped keeping track of them. Typically, such reports were about symptoms they had never before experienced until they started using aspartame-sweetened products, he noted.[42] (Back in 1996, we were told that 72 percent of the agency's total number of adverse reaction reports had been in regard to NutraSweet, a proprietary brand-name version of aspartame, since its introduction in 1980.[43])

Symptoms chronicled during that period alone provide a pretty good idea of the types of problems aspartame is capable of producing.

In an epidemiological survey that appeared in the *Journal of Applied Nutrition* back in 1988, the late Dr. H. J. Roberts, a diabetes specialist from Palm Beach, Florida, analyzed reactions from 551 affected individuals and found that the most common included headaches, dizziness, confusion and memory loss, severe drowsiness, eye problems such as decreased vision, blurring, bright flashes and tunnel vision, severe depression, anxiety attacks, and extreme irritability.

A smaller number of respondents suffered from auditory problems, including tinnitus, extreme noise intolerance, and hearing impairment, eye pain, pins and needles, convulsions and blackouts, slurring of speech, tremors, palpitations and rapid heartbeat, shortness of breath, nausea, diarrhea and abdominal pain, severe joint pain, restless leg syndrome, and various skin problems, including severe itching and hives. A few reported things like pain on swallowing, actual weight gain, low blood sugar attacks, bloating and fluid retention, burning on urination, thinning of hair, and, perhaps scariest of all, blindness in one or both eyes.[44] (Dr. Roberts went on to provide a detailed account of these reactions in a book more than one thousand pages long, which he called *Aspartame Disease: An Ignored Epidemic*, published in 2001.)

While the FDA might characterize such reports as "anecdotal," the fact that they're experienced first-hand rather than in a laboratory setting often makes them far more credible. In his book, *Excitoxins: The Taste that Kills*, neurosurgeon Dr. Russell Blaylock points out that many medical discoveries began with "anecdotal" accounts, and calls the tendency to dismiss them "poor science."

Blaylock cites examples of patients who suddenly developed grand mal seizures that seemed to correspond with the introduction of aspartame in their diet, as reported in 1985 by Dr. Richard J. Wurtman in the medical journal *Lancet*. One case in particular involved a fifty-four-year-old woman with no known medical problems who had been taking medication for depression for five years, when she suddenly experienced a grand mal seizure followed by a behavioral change marked by manic activity, agitation, and insomnia. What her doctors discovered was that just prior to that episode, she had started substituting NutraSweet for sugar in her tea, which she habitually drank in large quantities. Only four days after her medication was stopped and the NutraSweet eliminated, she lost the symptoms and had remained seizure-free when examined a year later.[45]

Perhaps it should come as no real surprise that thousands of people have reported such side effects, given that aspartame started life not as an artificial sweetener, but rather as a drug.

How politics superseded science to bring us to where we are today

It all began back in 1965 with a team of scientists employed by the pharmaceutical company G.D. Searle who were looking for a treatment for ulcers. One of them, James Schlatter, accidentally got a substance he was working with, called aspartylphenylalanine-methyl-ester—or aspartame—on his finger. Upon licking that same finger to pick up a piece of paper, or so the story goes, he took note of an unusually sweet taste. A further taste test revealed that it was indeed aspartame that was so finger-lickin' good. Forget about ulcers—serendipity had just resulted in the discovery of a new artificial sweetener estimated to "have a potency of 100–200 times sucrose . . . and to be devoid of unpleasant aftertaste."[46]

Before it could be introduced to the public, however, something further was required—approval from the FDA. That agency, it turned out, couldn't simply be sweet-talked into assenting to the marketing of aspartame as a food additive once some serious questions about its safety arose.

The first major red flag was raised by Dr. John Olney, a neuroscientist at Washington University in St. Louis, who discovered that the aspartic acid it contained produced holes in the brains of baby mice.[47] (Dr. Olney, in fact, made similar discoveries about monosodium glutamate (MSG), which ultimately resulted in its removal from baby food, and led to his categorizing both the free glutamate it contains and the aspartic acid in aspartame as "excitoxins" that can literally excite certain brain cells to death—a subject to be discussed in the chapter on MSG.)

Searle, however, conducted its own safety testing and, although one of its researchers confirmed Dr. Olney's findings, went ahead and sought the FDA's blessings based on what it claimed were a hundred studies. Despite an FDA scientist's opinion that the information provided by the company was "inadequate to permit an evaluation of the potential toxicity of aspartame," it managed to win provisional approval for the substance to be used in dry food. That is, until Olney and James S. Turner, a lawyer and consumer advocate who authored the 1970 landmark book, *The Chemical Feast*, submitted a petition challenging that decision. That resulted in a hearing before a public board of inquiry and a reexamination of those studies that found Searle had "manipulated its test data, and that its research techniques left a lot to be desired in the way of proficiency and accuracy."[48]

And that wasn't all. At the start of 1977, the FDA was so put off by these findings that, for the first time ever, it requested a grand jury investigation of whether Searle executives should be indicted for misrepresentation and for knowingly misrepresenting findings, "concealing material facts and making false statements." The probe was dropped after the US attorney involved in the case quit to take a job with Searle's law firm, delaying the proceedings long enough to put the charges beyond the statute of limitations.

In the meantime, however, FDA investigators, led by agent Jerome Bressler, went ahead with their own examination (known as the Bressler Report), which found just how many flaws existed in Searle's studies. It turned out, for example, that 98 of 196 animals died during one of them and autopsies were not done until much later—sometimes over a year later. In others, abnormalities had been found and not reported, including a mass, a uterine polyp, and ovarian neoplasms. There were even discrepancies in reports of whether a particular rat used in one study had lived or died.

Finally, in 1980, the public board of inquiry determined that it had "not been presented with proof of reasonable certainty that aspartame is safe for use as a food additive," and, perhaps scariest of all, that NutraSweet should be denied approval pending further research on whether it caused brain tumors. Concurring with that conclusion the following year were three of six in-house FDA scientists who analyzed the link between aspartame and brain tumors.[49]

Case closed, right? Well, not quite, because that corresponded with the time Ronald Reagan took office with promises of curtailing the powers of government regulators. On his transition team was none other than Donald Rumsfeld, later best known as George W. Bush's defense secretary, and then Searle's CEO. He apparently had a plan for making an end run around the opinion of those FDA scientists and getting NutraSweet on the market—one that involved choosing the next FDA commissioner himself. That was Dr. Arthur Hull Hayes, a Pennsylvania State University professor of medicine and Reagan appointee, who made giving NutraSweet the green light one of his first orders of business. (A little more than two years later, and shortly before aspartame was first introduced in diet soda, Hayes, in a classic example of the "revolving door" between government and industry, resigned from the FDA and took a job as senior scientific consultant for Burson-Marseller, the PR firm used by Searle. A number of FDA officials who worked under him were subsequently recruited by Searle or its successor, Monsanto.)[50]

That was that. Despite a further challenge mounted by Turner and another consumer advocate, Dr. Woodrow Monte, director of the Food Science and Nutritional Laboratories at Arizona State University,[51] aspartame (originally under the brand names NutraSweet and Equal) remained on the market as an officially approved food additive, eventually going from soft drinks into an estimated six thousand diet and sugar-free products[52] (even including children's vitamins). In 1985, Searle was purchased by chemical giant Monsanto (which has since reorganized as an agricultural company best known for the herbicide Roundup and the genetically engineered seeds that accommodate it), with NutraSweet becoming a separate subsidiary and its patent on aspartame subsequently expiring.

It was, as Turner later told us, a case of "that which had been won by a scientific process (being) lost to a political process."[53]

Just how much physiological damage that political process has resulted in has been the subject of considerable speculation ever since. Despite the FDA's attempts to dismiss all such reports as "anecdotal," however, many of them have been backed up by medical experts, such as Dr. Richard Wurtman, a leading neurologist and former head of clinical research at MIT, who testified before a US Senate Commission on NutraSweet's effects chaired by Ohio Senator Howard Metzenbaum. Wurtman told the panel that he believed that epileptic seizures and other symptoms exhibited by a few hundred patients following aspartame ingestion could be linked to the component phenylalanine, on which his lab had already conducted several hundred studies.[54]

Wurtman was not the only expert to have serious doubts about the safety of aspartame. According to French investigative journalist and author Marie-Monique Robin, a survey of sixty-seven scientists done around that time by the Government Accountability Office (GAO) at

Metzenbaum's request found that more than half had concerns about it, with a dozen voicing "serious concerns."[55]

Of particular concern to Metzenbaum were the effects of an aspartame breakdown component, diketopiperazine, or DKP, which some research has implicated in brain tumor development. The senator made a point of this in a 1986 letter to Utah Senator Orrin Hatch, chairman of the Labor and Human Resources Committee, seeking support for an inquiry, in which he noted that a key test on DKP that the FDA had originally told the Justice Department could require submission to the grand jury had never gotten such scrutiny. He also revealed how a Searle "strategy memo" had talked about getting the FDA into the "habit of saying yes" by first submitting safety issues "involving little or no breakdown of NutraSweet into DKP."[56]

Are non-caloric synthetic sweeteners contributing to obesity?

A growing body of scientific evidence has indicated that consumption of artificial sweeteners, such as aspartame, as a way of controlling weight may actually be counterproductive.

In 2014, an Israeli study points to artificial sweeteners as likely culprits in the development of "obesity-related metabolic conditions," such as type 2 diabetes, by interfering with our internal ecosystem of gut bacteria, which is an essential part of the body's mechanism for regulating blood sugar.

The study found that the three most widely used non-caloric synthetic sweeteners—saccharin, sucralose, and aspartame—actually raised blood sugar levels in mice by creating increased glucose intolerance. No such effect was observed in mice either drinking water by itself or water with plain sugar added to it, whether fed normal chow or a high-fat diet.

The researchers also did comparative testing on nearly four hundred non-diabetic individuals. They found those who consumed artificial sweeteners to have significantly altered gut bacteria, along with signs of glucose intolerance and raised blood sugar levels similar to the results found in the mice.

These findings suggested that "non-caloric artificial sweeteners may have directly contributed to enhancing the exact epidemic that they themselves were intended to fight," noted the
lead author, Dr. Eran Segal of the Weizmann Institute of Science.
He added that the results had convinced him to stop using artificial sweeteners in his coffee.[57]

In another more recent study of more than three thousand pregnant women and their infants a year after delivery,
researchers led by Meghan Azad, assistant professor in pediatrics and child health at University of Manitoba, found moms
who reported consuming more artificial sweeteners in beverages were twice as likely to have children that were overweight
or obese at one year as the ones who reported using them
less.[58]

Those brain tumors: more than merely rumors

"Incredible and unprecedented."

That was the phrase used by the late renowned neuroscientist
Dr. Olney to describe the incidence of brain tumors that occurred in
laboratory rats fed aspartame during Searle's own research.

Olney based that assessment on the results of seven studies involving
a total of 59,000 rats, only 0.08 percent of which developed "spontaneous" brain tumors. By contrast, he noted, the number of tumors that
occurred in the rats fed aspartame was forty-seven times higher. Even
allowing for a Searle estimate of brain tumors developing by themselves
in 0.15 percent of rats, the ones given aspartame still had twenty-five
times more.

Those figures became even more alarming once the ages of the rats
used in the research were factored in. Brain tumors, he pointed out, are
an extreme rarity before rats reach the age of one and a half, and usually
don't show up until after the age of two, which was the point when the
Searle study ended. In fact, a study of 41,000 rats detected none by 60
weeks and only one by 70 weeks. Yet Searle reported six brain tumors as
having developed in the aspartame-fed animals after 76 weeks. Although

the company claimed that the findings reflected how scrupulously it had searched the slides involved, as Dr. Blaylock points out, the tumors shown on slides were big enough to be seen with the naked eye, according to neuropathologists who examined them.

When confronted with these contrasting sets of figures, Searle went back to its laboratory and came up with some results that, according to Blaylock, "can only be characterized as bizarre," with brain tumors shown in both groups of rats at a rate thirty times higher than that considered normal for their spontaneous development.[59]

This extreme inconsistency is one that Blaylock attributes to what those FDA investigators found in 1975—evidence of "apparent irregularities in data collection and reporting practices that included sloppy lab work, clerical errors, mix-ups of experimental and control animals, "pathological specimens lost because of improper handling, and a variety of other errors" that, even if not intentional, "all conspire to obscure positive findings and produce falsely negative results."[60] In several instances, for example, Blaylock notes that the investigators found malignant tumors classified as benign and in others, tumors had been removed from rats and tissue slides and reported as normal."[61]

While those early indicators of a link between aspartame and brain tumors in lab rats doesn't prove it causes them in humans, Blaylock cites a two-thirds increase in brain tumors seen in people over 65 between 1973 and 1990.[62] And in the two decades between 1975 and 1995, the National Cancer Institute, looking into trends in childhood cancer and mortality, found a "statistically significant" rise in brain and other central nervous system cancers.[63]

Brain tumors, it turns out, aren't the only kinds of abnormal cell growths that may be linked to aspartame consumption. Other types of cancer have also been linked to the sweetener in rat studies, as the Center for Science in the Public Interest pointed out in a 2015 press release that urged pop star Taylor Swift to rethink her endorsement of Diet Coke in an ad campaign. "Scientists generally accept that if a chemical causes cancer in animals it likely increases the risk of cancer in humans," the release noted, adding that CSPI recommends that consumers avoid aspartame and has urged food manufacturers not to use it. The group's director, Michael Jacobson, also told the Grammy-winning singer (who has helped promote the work of anticancer charities) that "to the extent that your endorsement encourages them to begin drinking Diet Coke, or to drink more, your endorsement is likely increasing your fans' risk of cancer."[64]

Given how the FDA has chosen to dismiss any and all such information related to aspartame, however, it's easy to see how celebrities such as Swift can allow themselves to become its pitchmen.

Recent research links heart risk and diet soda consumption in older women

The notion that aspartame-laced diet soda is a healthy alternative to the so-called "sugary drinks" (which are actually sweetened with high fructose corn syrup, a badditive whose effects are discussed in a later chapter) is one that has persisted for many years, thanks in no small part to the FDA's dismissal of many thousands of consumer complaints as merely "anecdotal."

Less easily ignored are a couple of recent studies done by major universities on how aspartame might affect human subjects.

One was a 2014 analysis out of the University of Iowa, and presented at the American College of Cardiology's 63rd Annual Scientific Session in Washington, DC. It found that otherwise healthy postmenopausal women who down two or more diet soda or fruit drinks a day are 30 percent more likely to suffer a heart attack, stroke, or other cardiovascular "event" and 50 percent more likely to die as a result than those who seldom or never consume such beverages.

In reaching that conclusion, researchers analyzed diet drink consumption and cardiovascular health in almost 60,000 women participating in the Women's Health Initiative Observational Study. They also adjusted the data to account for demographic characteristics and other risk factors, including body mass index, smoking, hormone therapy use, physical activity, energy intake, salt intake, diabetes, hypertension, high cholesterol, and non-diet beverage intake.

The analysis also found that, on average, the subjects who consumed two or more diet drinks a day had a higher prevalence of diabetes, high blood pressure, and higher body mass index. Lead researcher Dr. Ankur Vyas, a fellow in cardiovascular disease at the university's hospitals and clinics, called the UI study one of the largest to be undertaken on this topic, and said its findings "are consistent with some previous data, especially those linking diet drinks to the metabolic syndrome."[65]

Another 2014 study performed at the University of North Dakota looked at the effects of aspartame consumption on healthy adults who consumed a high-aspartame diet for eight days followed by a low-aspartame diet for eight days, with a two-week period in between. When on the high-aspartame diet, participants were more irritable, exhibited more depression, and performed worse on spatial orientation tests. "Given that the higher intake level tested here was well below the maximum acceptable daily intake level of 40–50 mg/kg body weight/day," noted an abstract on the study, "careful consideration is warranted when consuming food products that may affect neurobehavioral health."[66]

Pushing petitioners aside

In a citizen petition he submitted to the FDA back in 2009, pediatrician Dr. K. Paul Stoller from Santa Fe, New Mexico, requested that the agency's approval of aspartame be revoked. The sweetener, he contended, "has been shown to be, and has always been known to be, a carcinogen" and therefore fell under the Delaney Clause, a section of the 1958 Food Additives amendment that prohibits the use of substances in food found to induce cancer in either humans or animals.

In support of that assertion, Stoller, who served as chief of hyperbaric medicine at the Amen Clinics, cited scientific research that included a 2007 long-term aspartame animal feeding study, published in *Environmental Health Perspectives*, in which "increases in total malignant tumors, lymphomas/leukemias, and mammary carcinomas were observed in male and/or female rats," including "statistically significant" increases in "lymphomas/leukemias in both male and female rats, mammary carcinomas in females, and tumor-bearing males."

The baby rats used in the study, Stoller noted, were exposed to aspartame both *in utero* and after weaning, whereas in an earlier study, the artificial sweetener was fed to rats once they were eight weeks old. The results of that one, he pointed out, included "statistically significant increased incidences of leukemias/lymphomas in both male and female rats," as well as "a few uncommonly occurring brain tumors" seen only in the aspartame-treated animals. The follow-up study, however, was far more robust, involving more animals and following them not only before birth, but for three years—equivalent to keeping tabs on people for eighty or ninety years.

However, Stoller's petition went well beyond such study results. It proceeded to review the whole corrupt history of the aspartame approval process, going back to the "fraudulent" research presented by G.D. Searle and the politics involved in getting aspartame past those public health hurdles, pointing out, for example, that despite three Congressional hearings from 1985 to 1987, "a senator linked with Monsanto made sure the bill to put a moratorium on aspartame and have [the National Institutes of Health] do independent studies on the problems being reported to the FDA never got out of committee."

Stoller also charged that the industry funded various groups, such as the American Diabetes Association, to push aspartame propaganda. According to Stoller, "full-time front groups" such as the Calorie Control Council (which claims that "unfounded allegations that aspartame is associated with a myriad of ailments . . . have continued to be spread via the Internet and the media by a few individuals who have no documented scientific or medical expertise"[67]) were being used to help manufacturers "keep pushing this poison," even while scientists looking into the toxic aspects of aspartame were being threatened. He disputed claims that most research has shown aspartame to be safe, pointing out that when Dr. Ralph Walton (who appeared on a *60 Minutes* segment about the sweetener) looked into the subject, he found that 92 percent of independent scientific peer-reviewed studies showed that there were problems with aspartame, "while only those funded or controlled by industry ever said it was safe."

As an example of what he called the "fraudulent" research used to prove aspartame's safety, Stoller contended that in one study "investigators were so worried somebody would have a seizure" that sixteen of the subjects were given antiseizure medication, and the amount of aspartame used was very small—a single capsule per day. "So when consumers complain of seizures they say, 'we did studies and aspartame doesn't cause seizures.'"[68]

Predictably, however, none of that cut any ice with the FDA. "Despite your many assertions, you have not identified any scientific data or other information that would cause the agency to alter its conclusions about the safety of aspartame," came the official response to Stoller's information-packed petition in October, 2014 from Steven Musser, Deputy Director for Scientific Operations of the Center for Food Safety and Applied Nutrition. Musser maintained that "regulatory authorities" around the world all agreed that "aspartame is safe for the general population except for individuals with phenylketonuria."

In addition to claiming that the FDA lacked a "full data set" for one of the studies Stoller cited, done by the European Ramazzini Foundation, Musser's letter went on to claim that its results were "compromised by significant shortcomings." However, in referring to the Bressler Report that was based on the agency's own investigation of the original flawed Searle studies, it came to the opposite conclusion. In that case, it found that "most of the shortcomings, transcription errors or changes in the study protocols were not of such magnitude that they would significantly alter the original conclusions of these studies."[69]

Apparently, maintaining a double standard poses no real problem for the FDA where research on aspartame is concerned. Stoller wasn't the only anti-aspartame activist to be stonewalled by the agency. Accompanying the rejection of his request was denial of yet another petition, this one filed back in 2002 by Dr. Betty Martini, founder of a Georgia-based nonprofit called Mission Possible World Health International, which sought to have "the neurotoxic drug, aspartame, masquerading as an additive" recalled, contending that it was responsible for a host of health problems, including seizures, tumors, and eye deterioration, as well as for being a "chemical hypersensitization agent" that interacts with many medications. (When several years elapsed during which Martini received no reply to her petition, which she charged should have been answered within 180 days, she filed an amendment in 2007 asking that it be banned as an "imminent health hazard.")

In turning down Martini's petition, Musser claimed it contained "anecdotal accounts of adverse effects of aspartame" and was lacking in "substantive scientific evidence demonstrating that aspartame's use presents a public health risk or that this sweetener is adulterated or misbranded" under the Federal Food, Drug, and Cosmetic Act. He also claimed that from 2004 through 2013 the Center for Food Safety had received just 195 reports of "adverse events" associated with aspartame consumption for which it could find "no causal link," nor did it know of "an established mechanism that would explain how aspartame is associated with the reported adverse events."

Musser did in fact contend that the FDA continues "to monitor the scientific literature for information that might indicate potential public health concerns" about aspartame, and would take "appropriate action" if it finds the sweetener's uses "do not meet the safety standards for food additives."[70]

That monitoring effort, however, appears to have missed an awful lot of scientific literature that not only already exists, but has been placed right before its eyes. But if the FDA has blinders on where aspartame safety is concerned, that's entirely understandable. For it to go back at this late date and acknowledge that approving aspartame all those years ago was a major blunder would substantially undermine public confidence in this regulatory agency's credibility.

The result has been what Dr. Roberts, in the introduction to his 2001 book, referred to as "a virtual blackout of information . . . about the adverse effects of aspartame," which has caused most physicians "to remain ignorant of aspartame disease or adamantly refuse to accept its legitimacy."[71] It's evident that little has changed since then, given the FDA's refusal to budge from its decades-old dismissal of the health hazards associated with this neurotoxic sweetener that were once acknowledged by its own investigators and scientists.

So maybe those who suffer from PKU are lucky in at least one respect: they've been officially warned away from aspartame, and have thus managed to avoid all its attendant risks and side effects. The rest of us, unfortunately, remain strictly on our own when it comes to steering clear of this pernicious drug that's been posing all these years as a healthy sweetener—and that continues to hide in so many innocent-looking foods and beverages.

Airline pilots on diet drinks: a disaster waiting to happen

We've all heard the recent news stories about airline pilots suspended for "flying under the influence." However, according to both activists working to collect real-life data on the effects of aspartame and a number of first-person accounts, the threat to airline passenger safety isn't just from pilots who have consumed alcoholic beverages prior to takeoff. It may also be from their drinking something as seemingly innocuous as diet soda, either before or during flights.

William R. Deagle, MD, a California-based holistic and integrative medicine practitioner who has worked as a civil aviation examiner, claims to have "personally examined pilots who suffered dangerous absence seizures (suspensions of consciousness that can last several seconds), blackout, and dangerous lack of judgment," all symptoms he says can occur for weeks after consuming the sweetener. According to Deagle, "it was an unwritten rule that aspartame was not to be used at the Air Force Academy," and most commercial pilots knew of the danger it posed years ago.[12]

Another medical expert, neurosurgeon Russell L. Blaylock, noted back in 2011 that he had reviewed some of the reports from airline and private pilots concerning adverse effects of aspartame and that "several of these complaints are related to the nervous system, which puts this in a category of great concern to the pilot as well as the general public. Some of the more common complaints include, disorientation, difficulty thinking and concentrating, visual blurring or even monocular blindness, seizures and heart failure."

Blaylock pointed out that elevated levels of two of aspartame's components, phenylalanine and aspartic acid, can significantly raise the risk of suffering a seizure, especially "if a diet drink is substituted for a meal," adding that "the combination of hypoglycemia and aspartame would also increase the likelihood of mental confusion and disorientation.

"In the pilot's situation," he warned, "this could be disastrous. It must be recognized that pilots would also be frequently exposed to other excitotoxins, such as MSG, hydrolyzed proteins, etc., that have a synergistic effect that greatly increases the likelihood of an adverse reaction."[73]

Such warnings, in fact, are similar to one that appeared back in 1992 in the US Air Force journal, *Flying Safety* (one extracted from an issue of *Navy Physiology*), which suggested that "a pilot who drinks diet sodas is more susceptible to flicker vertigo, or to flicker-induced epileptic activity," and "that ALL pilots are potential victims of sudden memory loss, dizziness during instrument flight and gradual loss of vision."[74] Other aviation journals also cautioned pilots about drinking aspartame-sweetened beverages around that period.

In a letter responding to the article in *Flying Safety*, Aspartame Consumer Safety Network founder Mary Nash Stoddard claimed that a Pilot Hotline set up by her organization for confidential reports of adverse reactions to aspartame had fielded over five hundred phone calls, some about incidents of grand mal seizures in the cockpits of commercial airliners.[75]

When we asked Blaylock whether consuming aspartame might also be a risk factor for train engineers, truck and bus drivers, or motorists, he replied, "It could be hazardous for these drivers under certain conditions—for instance it can induce severe hypoglycemia in those with reactive hypoglycemia and [in] those with a seizure potential it could precipitate a seizure."

All of this raises the question of whether diet drinks and other products containing aspartame might have played a role in some of the train and bus crashes that have been blamed on "human error." While we really can't say, the frightening potential that something as seemingly innocuous as a soft drink could bring about such a catastrophe can't be dismissed as long as this ill-conceived badditive remains on the market.

The saga of stevia: how industry and the FDA tried—and failed—to suppress a natural sweetener

The ambivalence of the FDA when it comes to food additives was never better demonstrated than in its contrasting attitudes toward aspartame and the sweet herb stevia.

Stevia, for the record, is the alternative sweetening agent that many people have now opted for in order to avoid both the calories of added sugar and the use of neurotoxic aspartame and other questionable artificial sweeteners. The leaves of this plant have been used for centuries by natives of parts of South America where it grows naturally. Stevia extracts became widely popular throughout much of the world during the twentieth century.

In addition to being naturally non-caloric, stevia is reputed to have various medicinal benefits—for example, it has been shown to help stabilize blood sugar and is actually beneficial to dental health. Perhaps best of all, unlike aspartame, there have never been any reported adverse effects from its use, and a series of extensive safety tests done some years ago by Japanese scientists found no health problems associated with it.

However, back in the early 1990s, stevia seemed to be public enemy number one. The FDA branded it as an "unsafe food additive" and imposed an "import alert," even going so far as to raid the warehouse of a stevia importer with federal marshals. Even though it gained some protection under the Dietary Supplement Health and Education Act of 1994, the agency did everything it could to hinder sales, restricting its use as an ingredient and prohibiting all mention of its sweetening ability.

What reportedly brought about this crackdown wasn't any consumer complaint, but reportedly a "trade complaint"—one originating from a firm the FDA never identified but that manufacturers of natural products claimed they were told was none other than the NutraSweet Company.

In acting on that complaint, the FDA characterized reams of information they had been given on stevia's long history of consumption as "anecdotal," and invoked a couple of studies in obscure journals that stevia might cause low blood sugar in people with hypoglycemia, which they admitted to us they hadn't actually seen.[76]

So, imagine how surprising it was for those of us who knew the whole story to suddenly see stevia appear in the supermarket alongside sugar and artificial sweeteners. What happened? How could this herb with the secret sweetness the FDA had spent so long trying to suppress suddenly emerge as the newest, no-calorie sweetener on the market?

To make a long story short, it seems that when enough consumers started looking for a natural alternative sweetener, the corporate world suddenly decided that stevia was something that might just prove profitable after all.

One of the first national stevia products to hit the shelf was PureVia, which submitted a notification to the FDA in May of 2008 saying it had "self" determined its stevia product to be "generally recognized as safe," or GRAS. The FDA issued a "no objection" letter later that year. So, how did PureVia succeed in a mission that even a very well-respected herbal association couldn't accomplish in the past? Maybe it was the economic clout behind the launching of the product, which was a joint effort of PepsiCo and another firm affiliated with Monsanto, the one-time corporate parent of NutraSweet (the same company that once reportedly tried to keep stevia off the market).

That's right—the aspartame people are now in the stevia business, with Merisant, a Monsanto spinoff formed in 2000, now giving "equal time" to the Equal brand of tabletop aspartame and PureVia Stevia.

The positive part of all this is that stevia is now much easier to find. However, not all those products are pure stevia extracts. Some are combined with cane sugar and others are bulked up with corn-derived ingredients. One, Cargill's Truvia, has had its claim to being "natural" challenged in a couple of lawsuits. While it contains a relatively small amount of stevia, its main ingredient, erythritol, was found in a Drexel University study to actually have insecticide-like effects on fruit flies.[77]

Such adulteration aside, the growing popularity of stevia despite all the obstacles put in its path by both industry and the FDA is an indication that as consumers grow more knowledgeable, the age of badditives in our food may be slowly drawing to a close.

Know your badditives and how to avoid them:

ASPARTAME

- Steer clear of any low-calorie or no-calorie beverages, including soda, flavored water, and tea.
- Be wary of "diet" or "low-cal" processed foods, especially products such as syrups, yogurt, puddings, and gelatin.
- Check before you chew! Practically every brand of gum out there uses an artificial sweetener, which is often aspartame.
- Be on the alert for notices on the labels of any food, beverage, or supplement that states it "contains phenylalanine" as a warning to those suffering from a condition called PKU. That means aspartame is one of the ingredients.
- Look for the presence of aspartame in vitamins and over-the-counter drugs. You might also ask the pharmacist if a prescription drug contains it, since, like other badditives, aspartame can show up in some surprising places.

BHA and BHT

From the Battlefield to Your Breakfast Table

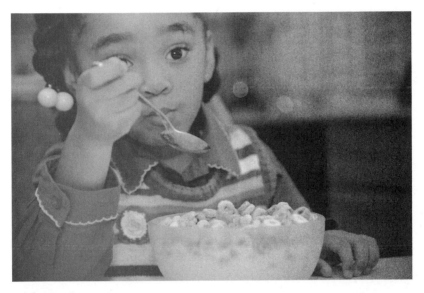

Credit: iStock

"Humans are not designed to eat petroleum—and when they do, bad things happen."

—Jane Hersey, national director,
Feingold Association of the United States

The industrial preservatives BHA (butylated hydroxyanisole) and BHT (butylated hydroxytoluene), like artificial colors, are derived from petroleum. So it should perhaps come as no surprise that these substances, which are used to give a wide range of processed food a longer shelf life, have also been the focus of behavioral and other health concerns, including cancer, for decades, even as the FDA has continued to declare them safe for use in food products (as well as medicines and cosmetics).

In fact, by adding this problematic pair to the list of ingredients he eliminated from the diets of kids being treating for attention deficit hyperactivity disorder (ADHD), Dr. Benjamin Feingold, the creator of the Feingold Program, saw the program's success rate rise from between 30 and 50 percent to 70 percent or more.[78]

How did this disreputable duo manage to slip into the food supply without causing the regulators to blink? Like other dubious developments—nerve gases adapted for use in pesticides, for example—they were products of the Second World War. Used to help keep combat soldiers' rations from going rancid, these chemicals needed to find a new market after the end of that conflict. That, according to the Feingold Association, is how they ended up "in foods, cleaning supplies, and plastics for a public enthralled with all things 'modern' and embracing of the idea of 'better living through chemistry.'"[79]

Maladjusted mice, problem children, and concerns over cancer

"Food is supposed to spoil eventually, but of course you want to eat it before it does," observes the Feingold Association's Jane Hersey. "These preservatives give food the appearance of being fresh—but it also doesn't take much of them to trigger serious health and behavioral problems in sensitive individuals."[80]

The latter concerns should certainly come as no big surprise, given that both BHA and BHT, which are banned in Japan and most European countries, have long been known to alter brain chemistry in mice exposed before birth. Back in 1974, researchers discovered that including 5 percent BHA or BHT in the diet of pregnant mice caused "a variety of behavioral changes" in their offspring. The baby mice exposed to BHA were slower learners and slept and groomed themselves less than control mice, while those given BHT, besides getting less sleep and showing decreased learning ability, also exhibited increased aggression.[81]

In addition to behavioral and nervous system effects, however, the Feingold Association points out that these particular preservatives have been shown to be "toxic to various cells and organs," to promote tumor growth, to weaken the immune system, and to have negative effects on reproduction. The fact that they are often used together in products is also bad news, since BHA can amplify the toxicity of BHT in your lungs, according to one study.[82]

Both preservatives, in fact, have been implicated as suspects in cancer formation. A University of Colorado study in 1989, for instance, found that BHT "can enhance the formation of carcinogen-induced lung tumors in mice."[83] BHA has also been repeatedly described in the National Toxicology Program's Annual Report on Carcinogens (cancer-causing agents) as "reasonably anticipated to be a human carcinogen" based on animal studies. In fact, when added to the diets of rats, mice, and hamsters, BHA resulted in both cancerous and noncancerous tumors,[84] and is on the state of California's list of "known carcinogens and reproductive toxicants."[85] Yet it has continued to be given GRAS (generally recognized as safe) status by the FDA despite the supposed prohibition on cancer-causing additives established by the Delaney Clause.

As if all that wasn't enough, BHT has been placed on The Endocrine Disruption Exchange (TEDX) List of Potential Endocrine Disruptors,[86] based on a study done in 2000 at the school of Biosciences at Britain's University of Birmingham.[87]

tBHQ: An artificial preservative currently suspected of causing food allergies

What turns a food additive into a badditive? It could be either of two things—when it is directly associated with various adverse reactions, or when research points to long-term health effects (or, sometimes, both).

It's that second character test that could well put a relative of BHA and BHT on the official badditive roster, too. The ingredient in question, tert-Butylhydroquinone or tBHQ, is another petroleum-based preservative used in processed foods ranging from cooking oil to candy (such as Reese's Peanut Butter Cups), which was given FDA approval back in 1972.

Unlike those other two preservatives, tBHQ had received relatively little attention that would have justified its being put in the same category as the rest of the badditives discussed in these pages. However, at the writing of this book, dramatic new research has emerged that could be a reason for consumers to make a point of avoiding it as well.

In July 2016, Michigan State University announced that Cheryl Rockwell, an assistant professor of pharmacology and toxicology at the College of Human Medicine, was investigating a possible link between tBHQ and the recent rise in food allergies.

Rockwell's research, which she has been conducting for the past nine years, has convinced her that tBHQ causes T cells, a key component of the body's immune system, to release proteins capable of triggering allergies to such foods as nuts, eggs, milk, wheat, and shellfish.

In a laboratory setting, she discovered that tBHQ caused T cells to behave differently than they ordinarily do. "The T cells stopped acting as soldiers in the defense against pathogens and started causing allergies," Rockwell said. That finding may indicate why a rise in food allergies and an increase in the severity of such reactions has corresponded with the amplified use of tBHQ. Rockwell's work in this area has been solid enough to win her an award from the National Institute of Environmental Health Sciences, along with a $1.5 million, five-year research grant.[88]

An object lesson in the power of consumers to bring about change

It wasn't until popular consumer advocate Vani Hara, known as the "Food Babe," posted an online petition signed by thousands of her followers calling on cereal giants Kellogg's and General Mills to stop using BHT, that any serious steps were taken by industry to curtail its use. Citing concerns expressed by both the Environmental Working Group and the

Center for Science in the Public Interest, she pointed out that European versions of some of the top-selling cereals made by these companies don't contain BHT, proving that it's not an essential ingredient, and asked why Americans should "needlessly consume a controversial chemical if these companies have already figured out how to make their cereals without it?"[89] Not long afterward, in early 2015, both General Mills and Kellogg's announced plans to replace it. Not that either company would acknowledge that Hari deserved the credit or that "food safety" has anything to do with that decision, however. A General Mills media relations manager was quoted as saying the company was "well down the path of removing it from our cereals . . . not for safety reasons, but because we think consumers will embrace it," while a spokesperson for Kellogg's maintained that the company has been in the process of "actively testing" natural alternatives to BHT "to ensure the same flavor and freshness," adding, "we know some people are looking for options without BHT."[90]

That's hardly surprising, given the reluctance of food manufacturers to acknowledge that long used ingredients may have been harmful or inadvisable. What is important is that it once again demonstrates the power of informed consumers to influence how food products are manufactured in a way that researchers can't and regulators for the most part won't.

Know your badditives and how to avoid them:

BHA and BHT

- Keep in mind that any non-organic processed food that contains fats or oils may also contain BHA or BHT—and always check the ingredients label (not the Nutrition Facts panel) for the presence of these preservatives.
- Don't just rely on a promise from a manufacturer to eliminate these preservatives from their products, since this takes time to accomplish. It's still best to do an ingredient label scan before putting any breakfast cereals into your shopping cart.
- Buy organic versions of processed items like cereals, baked goods, and snack foods whenever possible.

CARRAGEENAN

The Thickener That's a Sickener

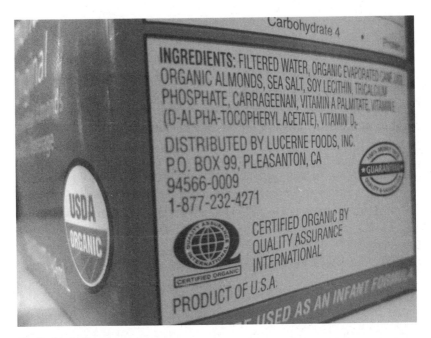

Credit: Linda Bonvie

"Putting carrageenan in food is like putting poison ivy in skin lotion. The only difference is we cannot see the inflammation, lesions, ulcerations, and polyps in our intestines. Both are natural, and both are cause for concern."
　　　　—Cornucopia Institute, updated report on carrageenan

Judging from the number of commercials on television for drugs designed to relieve various gastrointestinal ills, one can easily conclude that millions of Americans are afflicted with a variety of such problems, ranging from bloating and discomfort to serious conditions such as irritable bowel syndrome and ulcerative colitis.

Could it be, however, that many of these maladies are the result of a single badditive, one that's long been considered so safe by virtue of being "natural" that it's even allowed in organic food, despite a growing body of scientific evidence that it's anything but?

The answer is a resounding "yes." If you're among those who suffer from chronic stomach issues, it's quite possible that they might be alleviated simply by removing from your diet any processed foods that contain the ingredient carrageenan, as has been attested to by some of those who have done just that (see box on page 50).

Carrageenan is used in a wide variety of processed foods and beverages, ranging from coconut water, low-fat dairy products, and dairy substitutes to nutrition bars, deli meats, and precooked chicken. It serves as a thickening agent, giving food a nice texture and fatty "mouth feel."

However, this tasteless, non-nutritive seaweed derivative has long been shown to cause harmful gastrointestinal inflammation and intestinal lesions.

It can also be replaced with safer ingredients that serve similar purposes, such as guar gum (which FDA researchers back in 1988 found did not produce colon damage in lab rats, whereas carrageenan did[91]). In some instances, all it takes to achieve the same effect is simply to shake a product's container before consuming its contents. Yet carrageenan continues to be used by many food companies, including some that claim to have only "healthy" ingredients in their products.

The official dismissal of a gut-wrenching "rap sheet"

Concerns about the safety of carrageenan date all the way back to 1969, when researchers linked its use in food to gastrointestinal disease and colon cancer in laboratory animals.

In 2013, The Cornucopia Institute, a non-profit farm policy research group based in Wisconsin, detailed the scientific studies and other evidence against this ingredient in a report titled *Carrageenan: How a "Natural" Food Additive Is Making Us Sick*, which strongly urges consumers to avoid foods containing it. The report noted that "[f]or individuals who consume carrageenan on a regular or daily basis, the inflammation will be prolonged and constant, which is a serious health concern since prolonged inflammation is a precursor to more serious disease," and pointed out that there are over one hundred human diseases, including cancer, associated with such constant inflammation.[92]

The Institute also sent a letter to then-FDA Commissioner Margaret Hamburg requesting reconsideration of a citizen petition filed in 2008 that asked the FDA to ban the use of carrageenan in food, which was turned down by the agency in 2012. The petition had been submitted by Dr. Joanne Tobacman, a physician-scientist at the University of Illinois at Chicago, who had spent almost two decades studying the effects of this additive and published eighteen peer-reviewed papers on the subject.

"When a body of publicly funded scientific literature points to harm from consuming a common, widely used yet unnecessary food ingredient, the FDA should act in the interest of public health," said the letter, which was signed by Charlotte Vallaeys, the Institute's Farm and Food Policy Director, who noted that every claim that supports the safety of carrageenan in foods and beverages "can be refuted, based on strong scientific evidence."

Her letter also included an appendix of studies that were both favorable and unfavorable to the petition, pointing out that those supporting it were funded by public and private institutions with no financial interest in the outcome, whereas the ones that didn't were "almost exclusively funded by the industry that profits from the continued use of carrageenan in food."

The letter further noted that "there are no benefits to society or public health from adding carrageenan to foods or beverages," which is done "solely to change the texture of food."[93]

As in so many other cases involving entrenched food additives, the FDA declined to act on that request. Undeterred, in April of 2016, The Cornucopia Institute came out with an updated forty-nine-page carrageenan report bearing the subtitle *New Studies Reinforce Link to Inflammation, Cancer and Diabetes*, which includes detailed summaries of scientific findings from 1969 through 2016, charts and graphs on technical issues, consumer responses related to carrageenan and gastro-intestinal symptoms, and even a section devoted to food manufacturers' responses to scientific data about carrageenan.

In other words, this is more than merely a superficial evaluation. As you read through it, you soon realize that the staffers of the Institute have really done their homework on this issue and put together what you might call a gut-wrenching "rap sheet" that should be setting off regulatory alarm bells. As of this writing, however, their efforts and expertise appear to have made not one iota of difference to the FDA's policymakers, who, as other instances chronicled in this book demonstrate, are seldom known to declare a food additive they have previously approved to be unsafe and order its removal.

Carrageenan, as the latest report notes, comes from red seaweed and can be processed into either what's called "food grade" or "degraded" varieties. Degraded carrageenan, recognized as a "possible human carcinogen," is not permitted in food by virtue of being extremely inflammatory—so much so that it has been extensively used in scientific studies to induce inflammation in laboratory animals in order to test certain drugs.

While "food grade" certainly sounds safe enough, numerous studies have shown even small levels of this version, which is commonly added to food products, are enough to cause inflammation in the human colon as well. That, the report claims, is due to carrageenan having "unique chemical bonds not found in other seaweeds or gums" that have been found to trigger an immune response in the body similar to that caused by pathogens like *Salmonella*, which in turn causes inflammation of the digestive tract. And prolonged inflammation, it points out, can lead to other serious disease, including cancer.[94]

Perhaps most disturbing, however, are findings that "food grade" carrageenan isn't really the harmless product it's cracked up to be. For one thing, none of the samples analyzed by six different laboratories at the request of the European Commission were entirely free of the degraded version considered to be a cancer risk, with one lab reporting that two-thirds of its samples had in excess of 5 percent (the highest amount found in a sample being 25 percent). For another, studies that simulated the acidic conditions in the human gastrointestinal tract found that food-grade carrageenan could be converted into the "degraded" variety through the process of digestion.[95]

A blot on the organic industry's reputation

What may be the worst aspect of all this is the continued permitted use of carrageenan in organic foods, which, as the Institute observes in its latest report, "should be a safe haven from harmful ingredients," as required by the Organic Foods Production Act of 1990. In addition to requiring that nonagricultural ingredients be determined safe to human health and not deleterious to the environment before they can be added to organic foods, that law also states that whatever nonorganic ingredients are used must be essential to producing food, which carrageenan isn't, since innocuous alternatives like locust bean gum and guar gum can be substituted for it.

"Yet carrageenan, a nonorganic, nonagricultural ingredient made its way into organic foods due to carelessness by government regulators, misinformation supplied by corporate 'independent' scientists advising the USDA, and successful lobbying by carrageenan manufacturers and food processors," the report contends.[96]

Back in 2012, the National Organic Standards Board (NOSB), a group that determines what nonorganic ingredients can be used in organic foods, approved, by a one-vote margin, the continued use of carrageenan in foods labeled as certified organic.

This NOSB stamp of approval, according to the Cornucopia Institute, has been the result of food industry executives and lobbyists having used persuasion tactics that "have become increasingly more manipulative and ethically questionable, as it becomes clear that scientific evidence is not on their side."[97] In past reviews, including the Sunset Review by the NOSB in 2012, the Institute contends that "lobbyists convinced enough corporate-friendly NOSB members, including employees of Whole Foods, Organic Valley, and Driscoll's, to ignore the disturbing findings of dozens of independently funded and peer-reviewed studies, including several that found higher rates of colon cancer in lab animals given a diet containing food-grade carrageenan."[98]

The Institute's most recent report also notes that the National Organics Program has stopped publishing the names of authors of technical reviews, so that it is "no longer possible . . . to scrutinize the backgrounds or qualifications of the scientists preparing these briefings for the NOSB members," which has resulted in a number of conflicts of interest being identified in the past.[99]

So, if the FDA refuses to budge, despite being presented with so much independent research that this thickener is a sickener, and even the NOSB can't muster a majority of its members to recognize that carrageenan is the sort of ingredient that has no business in organic foods, what incentive do food processors have to remove it?

The answer is: the incentive that you, the consumer, provides them by refusing to spend your money on products that contain it and purchasing those that don't instead.

How eliminating carrageenan from their diets has changed some people's lives

To get an idea of just how disruptive to the digestive system carrageenan can be, you need look no further than the "Consumer Responses: Carrageenan & GI Symptoms" section in the Cornucopia Institute's latest report on this ingredient and its effects.

In response to an online survey posted by the Institute over a three-year period, some 1,397 individuals reported either that their gastrointestinal symptoms had completely disappeared or greatly improved after giving up foods containing carrageenan.

A resident from Manitoba, Canada, for example, describes having suffered "tremendous stomach cramps, body aches, and extreme bloating" lasting from twenty-four to forty-eight hours after eating various foods. She then discovered from a food journal that these foods all contained carrageenan. Since removing carrageenan from her diet, she said, the problems stopped; however, she noted that she had to be very careful not to ingest even the smallest amount, as it will cause her "hours of suffering."

Another respondent from Morgantown, West Virginia, tells of "nonstop throwing up and sweats/chills," visits to the emergency room, needing fluids and medication, and becoming severely dehydrated. All tests failed to find a cause except one, which involved a barium drink containing carrageenan. When the drink caused profuse vomiting, she realized that the ingredient was the probable cause.

Then there's the St. Louis resident who describes having gastrointestinal pain that "would literally incapacitate" her after consuming ice cream and coffee shop smoothies, though she was not lactose intolerant. After noticing that all the products involved had carrageenan in common, she started avoiding the additive and is now able to do things she couldn't do previously, such as going on overnight camping and canoeing trips.

As a woman from Ottawa, Canada, puts it, "Now that I have eliminated carrageenan from my diet, I can finally lead a normal life."[100]

A carrageenan about-face that shows how consumers can ultimately call the shots

As the Cornucopia Institute pointed out in its letter to the FDA, some food manufacturers are already replacing carrageenan with other thickeners and stabilizers, or eliminating thickeners altogether and asking their customers to shake the product before consumption. "If carrageenan is prohibited, the food industry will quickly adapt," it maintained. In some cases, that appears to be exactly what's taking place—with pressure from enlightened consumers serving as the catalyst for change.

A perfect illustration of this is the 180-degree turnaround done by WhiteWave Foods, whose brands include Horizon and Silk. The company's resistance to any suggestion that carrageenan be removed from its products is chronicled in the Institute's initial 2013 report, which tells how consumers who posted their concerns on Horizon Organic's Facebook wall were assured that food-grade carrageenan was safe. When these consumers replied that scientific studies showed otherwise, they were given a perfunctory response about how the company was "always monitoring and reviewing emerging science." Furthermore, the report noted, the company's vice president and chief lobbyist, despite being among those provided the latest scientific findings about the additive's harmful effects, ended up testifying in favor of keeping it in organic foods at the 2012 NOSB meeting.[101]

However, after "Food Babe" Vani Hari alerted the followers of her popular blog to the dangers of carrageenan,[102] WhiteWave totally reversed gears and announced plans in 2014 to phase it out of their brands, noting, "Our consumers have expressed a desire for products without it and we are listening!" The Associated Press quoted company spokeswoman Sara Loveday as stating that WhiteWave "still thinks carrageenan is safe, but decided to remove it because customer feedback has been so strong," adding, "When you get to a certain point of how vocal and strongly a consumer feels about it, we felt it was time to make a change."[103]

Apparently, then, such feedback is what's really required to get this inflammatory additive and other pernicious ingredients out of our food. That begins with reading the ingredients label on products (even organic ones, where carrageenan is concerned), avoiding those with harmful additives, and letting the manufacturers of those foods know the reason why.

How to keep carrageenan out of your best friend's diet

Since carrageenan has remained in so many "people foods," despite all the studies linking it to damage to the gastrointestinal system, it should come as no surprise that it's also present in quite a number of canned pet foods—especially those made for cats.

Finding high-quality canned cat foods that don't contain this red flag ingredient can sometimes be a bit difficult. But if you want to keep Fluffy happy and purring and perhaps spare yourself and her unnecessary visits to the vet, there are some carrageenan-free products now being offered by pet-supply stores (such as Wild Calling and Nutro FreeStyle brands), as well as others that can be ordered online.

Unless a product is advertised as being "carrageenan-free," however, it's always best to check the ingredients before purchasing it (just as with "people food"), since this ingredient is often hidden among more beneficial ones.

Know your badditives and how to avoid them:

CARRAGEENAN

- Since carrageenan, unfortunately, can be found in a lot of so-called "healthy" foods, including organic ones, reading ingredient labels is one of the only ways to be sure you're not ingesting it.
- Be especially careful when buying products such as almond, soy, and rice beverages, coconut water, and even ice cream.
- Look for carrageenan-free pet foods. Most brands of canned cat food in particular seem to contain the additive (and if you own a cat you know that they can be particularly prone to digestive issues). Beware of "pate" or loaf-type foods, as these are the ones where you're most likely to find it.

FLUORIDE

Hazardous Waste in Our Water That Ends up in Our Food

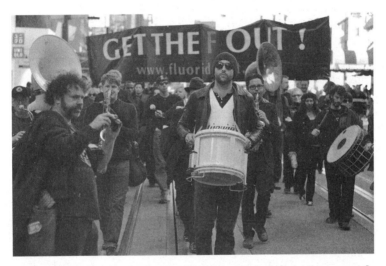

Even though San Francisco, like many other cities, has had its drinking water fluoridated for decades, residents continue to demand that this toxic substance be removed from a water supply that originates from the pristine melting snows of Yosemite National Park. *Credit: miker / Shutterstock.com*

"The face-lift performed on fluoride more than fifty years ago has fooled a lot of people. Instead of conjuring up the image of a crippled worker or a poisoned forest, we see smiling children. Fluoride's ugly side has almost entirely escaped the public gaze. . . . Yet, we are exposed to fluoride from more sources than ever. We consume the chemical from water and toothpaste, as well as from processed foods made with fluoridated water and fluoride-containing chemicals."
—Christopher Bryson, *The Fluoride Deception*

What better, healthier way to start the day than with a steaming bowl of organic oatmeal, sweetened with organic honey and maybe topped with some organic strawberries? What could possibly be wrong with that?

Well, how about the addition of a small amount of hazardous industrial waste?

We know—it probably sounds ridiculous. Where would such an unlikely toxic badditive even come from? The oats? The honey? The strawberries that are supposed to have been grown in a chemical-free environment?

The answer is: none of the above, but rather the water from your kitchen faucet you used to make the oatmeal. The same water that you may have taken the precaution of filtering against contaminants.

But then, this particular contaminant isn't one that's there by accident, as so many forms of water pollution are. Rather, it's been deliberately added in many locales for many years, in amounts ranging from 0.7 to 1.2 parts per million (ppm) for the purported purpose of protecting your children's teeth against cavities.

It's fluoride, a toxic substance once used to poison roaches and rodents—and it's something the Environmental Protection Agency has assigned a maximum contaminant level (MCL) for drinking water of 4 ppm, above which it can cause "skeletal damage,"[104] although that level, according to critics, was actually set way too high for children. (An advisory panel appointed by the Surgeon General's office in 1982 recommended by a vote of 10 to 2 that MCL for children up to age nine be set between 1.4 and 2.4 ppm, but the EPA opted to set it at 4 ppm, according to former EPA scientists Robert Carton, who called it an example of political interference with science.)[105]

Instead, it's sold to municipalities across the US to *add* to the water that comes out of your tap. Removing it requires a special water filter—not the kind you would ordinarily buy from your home supply center or supermarket.

But isn't fluoride something your dentist recommends—a substance found in most toothpastes and mouthwashes? How could it be that bad if the government actually encourages locales to put it in the water?

The answer is intertwined with intrigue. What if we told you that it was precisely *because* fluoride is so toxic that it ultimately ended up becoming an added ingredient in our water, and, in turn, in various foods and beverages? In fact, it appears that the original purpose of adding fluoride really wasn't to protect children's teeth; instead, it was a question of "national security," that is, to shield our nuclear weapons program—as well as a number of major industries—from liability for damage that this toxic substance was causing to people's health and properties.

Admittedly, that may sound rather perverse and more than a little bizarre, which may be one reason you're not hearing it from major media outlets. However, the records that substantiate this claim would be hard to refute.

The "F" files

"Something is burning up the peach crops around here."

That was how one aspect of a strange and frightening phenomenon that occurred in the southwestern part of New Jersey during the summer of 1943 was described. Reports from farmers in an area bordering the Delaware River also included accounts of dead poultry, sick horses, crippled cows, and illnesses among farm workers after eating produce they had just picked.[106]

The implications of those reports, along with lawsuits that resulted after the Second World War had ended, would resonate profoundly within the US government and military. That's because what was at stake was nothing less than the country's ability to continue with its nuclear weapons program without concerns about public safety being raised. The events that followed are chronicled in an extensively documented article written in 1997 by investigative journalists Christopher Bryson and Joel Griffiths entitled, "Fluoride, Teeth and the Atomic Bomb." The authors had spent a year researching the article but were unable to get it published in *The Christian Science Monitor*, which had commissioned it, despite favorable comments from editors.[107] (The article, now available online, was included in the following year's "Project Censored" series, which focuses on important news stories that have been neglected by mainstream media. According to the authors, at least a dozen media outlets here and in the UK "expressed strong interest" in running it, but all later declined. "The facts were never in question," they added, and there are 155 pages of supporting documentation.)[108]

As Bryson and Griffiths discovered in the course of their research, the damage to those Garden State farms, which were known for their high-quality peaches and tomatoes, and to their occupants was due to contamination from the fluoride produced by a nearby du Pont plant for the top-secret Manhattan Project. Large quantities of fluoride, it turned out, were essential in processing the uranium and plutonium needed to manufacture atomic bombs. And, in the opinion of those charged with assembling an arsenal of such weapons, something had to be done to counteract any potential adverse publicity that might result if that information ever became public knowledge.

Thus was born the practice of adding fluoride to drinking water for the purported purpose of helping to prevent cavities—a solution to a legal and public relations dilemma that would probably have never gotten off the drawing board had its details not been kept strictly confidential. (It's interesting to note that the original idea of fluoridation resulted from reports that people with "mottled enamel"—actually dental fluorosis—due to high amounts of naturally occurring fluoride in their water also had decay-resistant teeth. According to the American Dental Association (ADA), during the 1930s, Dr. H. Trendley Dean, a dental officer of the US Public Health Service, and his associates "had made the critical discovery that fluoride levels of up to 1.0 part per million (ppm) in the drinking water *did not cause the more severe forms of dental fluorosis.*"[109])

After first successfully persuading the FDA not to pursue its own probe of the New Jersey contamination episode, as well as sweet-talking and stonewalling the farmers bringing the litigation (which eventually was settled for token amounts of money), key figures in atomic bomb development undertook their own top-secret review of fluoride safety. Program F, as it was code-named, was initiated at the University of Rochester, where key atomic bomb research was conducted both during and after the war. Its main purpose, according to declassified documents from the era, was to bolster the government's defense in any further fluoride-related litigation.

Such documentary evidence, noted Jacqueline Kittrell, a Tennessee public interest lawyer specializing in nuclear cases, indicated that the university's research on fluoride stemmed from the New Jersey lawsuits and "was performed in anticipation of lawsuits against the bomb program for human injury." Studies of this sort, she added, "would not be considered scientifically acceptable today because of their inherent bias to prove the chemical safe."[110]

However, Program F wasn't simply based on laboratory experiments. As the declassified documents uncovered by Bryson and Griffiths showed, it ultimately involved turning the unsuspecting residents of the city of Newburgh, New York, into human guinea pigs by deliberately adding sodium fluoride to their water supply (and supposedly comparing the resulting statistics from those in nearby Kingston). Chairing the committee that had proposed this operation was Dr. Harold C. Hodge, who earlier had been chief of fluoride toxicology studies for the University of Rochester's participation in the Manhattan Project.

Over the following decade, "Newburgh Demonstration Project" administrators, assisted by state department of health personnel, secretly collected and examined blood and tissue samples from local residents. According to the two investigative journalists, "Health Department personnel cooperated, shipping blood and placenta samples to the Program F team at the University of Rochester." Those studies also helped determine what levels of fluoride could be tolerated by people exposed to it during the building of nuclear weapons.

Finally, in 1956, a report was issued proclaiming that this toxic substance was safe for Americans in "small concentrations," with Dr. Hodge himself offering biological proof "based on work performed . . . at the University of Rochester Atomic Energy Project."

That report, interestingly enough, was published in the *Journal of the American Dental Association*, the same professional journal in which a heavily censored version of a study of factory workers engaged in fluoride production for atomic bombs had appeared eight years earlier. Only when the journalists compared the published rendition of that study with the original did they discover some glaring omissions. For example, the fact that most of the workers had lost their teeth, that they had to wear rubber boots due to the fluoride fumes disintegrating the nails in their shoes, and that fluoride exposure may have had a similar effect on their teeth. Instead, the published article reported that the men simply had fewer cavities and that they were "unusually healthy, judged from a medical and dental point of view."

Bolstered by conclusions that, in retrospect, were highly suspect and steeped in conflict of interest, water fluoridation would subsequently proceed to go nationwide. But upon learning of the revelations uncovered by Bryson and Griffiths about the role unwittingly played by the people of Newburgh, then-Mayor Audrey Carey, who recalled having had her own teeth and "a peculiar fusion of two finger bones on her left hand" examined by fluoridation project doctors at a local health clinic, likened what had taken place there to the notorious experiments done on syphilis patients in Tuskegee, Alabama.[111]

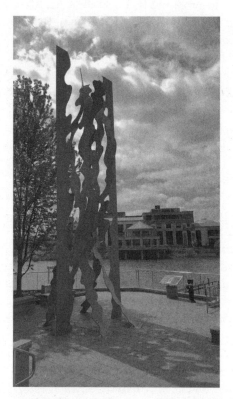

Steel Water is the name of an abstract sculpture commissioned by the West Michigan Dental Community to commemorate the role of Grand Rapids as the nation's first city to have its water supply fluoridated in 1945. Designed by the late Dutch artist Cyril Lixenberg and installed in 2007, it has an accompanying plaque that gushes effusively over the purported importance of fluoridation in "restoring good oral health for our nation and indeed the world," without mentioning that most of the world has since rejected the practice. *Credit: Lesley Ann, The Offbeat Path*

Newburgh, however, wasn't the first community to have sodium fluoride experimentally added to its water supply. That distinction belongs to Grand Rapids, Michigan, where the first fluoridation "demonstration project" began a few months earlier in January, 1945. The stated intent at the time was to compare the occurrence of cavities in children's teeth with those of nearby Muskegon, which was to remain unfluoridated for the next fifteen years.

That's not quite the way it worked out, however. After only five years, tooth decay rates declined in both cities, and the experiment was ended by having fluoride added to Muskegon's water as well. When data from this aborted "trial" was analyzed by a team of statisticians, it determined that "the lack of sophistication shown in selecting the sample leads to complete bewilderment as to the precise effects or the extent of the effect of fluoridation."[112]

How fluoridation's initial critics inadvertently helped promote it

Government officials, of course, couldn't have embarked on their pro-fluoridation propaganda program of the post-war years without a little help from their friends in the industrial sector. In fact, the stage had already been set for this effort back in the 1930s, when fluoride producers and users—and aluminum manufacturers in particular—became increasingly alarmed about reports of its toxic effects on workers and lawsuits from farmers whose cattle had been poisoned in the vicinity of smelters. As chronicled by Bryson in his 2004 book, *The Fluoride Deception,* they solicited the help of Gerald Cox, a Mellon Institute scientist engaged in research on tooth decay in making this industrial poison and source of water contamination out to be a kind of miraculous dental health discovery.[113]

Oddly enough, the early critics of fluoridation, most notably The John Birch Society and other groups considered to be right-wing extremists, were convinced that it was all a plot that originated in the Soviet Union. This view of the practice was actually the prototype for the "conspiracy theory"—a label that industry and its boosters in media now conveniently attach to any and all attempts to expose products and processes that pose a threat to public health (see box).

The movie mockery that made further inquiry politically incorrect

Anyone who's ever seen the 1964 black comedy *Dr. Strangelove* will remember the absurdly humorous depiction of the deranged General Jack Ripper, who takes it upon himself to launch a nuclear attack on the then–Soviet Union. In a memorable scene, Ripper explains his motive to a bewildered British officer as being "to stop an international communist conspiracy" from attempting to "sap and impurify all of our precious bodily fluids" by "introducing a foreign substance" into them. "Do you realize," he exclaims, "that fluoridation is the most monstrously conceived and dangerous Communist plot we have ever had to face?"

The character of General Ripper, of course, was based on people who actually voiced such ideas, and were often referred to as being on society's "lunatic fringe." Making a mockery of them in a movie, however, had the effect of helping stifle any legitimate debate about the advisability of adding fluoride to drinking water for many years by subjecting anyone who opposed fluoridation to scorn and ridicule.

As enlightened as they were, the moviemakers may have been as much in the dark as most other people were about the secret history of fluoridation. As Christopher Bryson noted in the introduction to his book, *The Fluoride Deception*, Nile Southern, the son of that film's screenwriter, Terry Southern, has since remarked that both his father and Stanley Kubrick, who cowrote, produced, and directed it, "would have been horrified" had they known that it was actually the work of US military and industrial interests.[114]

Such "lunacy by association" gave advocates of fluoridating tap water free rein to continue the program throughout the country without having to contend with any meaningful doubts, questions or criticism.

While their idea that fluoridation was all a plot hatched by the Russians may have been absurd, those initial opponents were correct in one respect. They accurately assessed how hazardous it was to our health—a realization that many scientists would eventually come to as well, although not until a couple of decades had passed. By that time, approximately two-thirds of the nation's population was drinking fluoridated water, not to mention consuming things like soup and juices that also contained it. (As it turned out, the probability that fluoride was neurotoxic was already known to some of the scientists affiliated with the Manhattan Project. That much is evident from a then "secret" memo received by its medical section chief, which mentions "a rather marked central nervous system effect" from uranium hexafluoride, whose "causative factor" was believed to be the fluoride component.[115])

Confirmation of that would come half a century later, in the form of peer-reviewed research done in the mid-1990s. One study indicated fluoride could accumulate in brain tissue, which, according to Dr. Phyllis Mullenix, a noted researcher on the subject with a PhD in pharmacology, could translate into cognitive problems in humans. A related study, she said, found that test animals given one part per million of fluoride in their drinking water—about the same amount then being added to municipal water supplies—suffered both brain and kidney damage. It also indicated that fluoride raised aluminum levels in the brain, raising concerns about a possible link to Alzheimer's (see the earlier chapter on aluminum).

Perhaps most frightening were the results of a study in which Mullenix took part, which was jointly sponsored by several highly reputable institutions, including divisions of Boston Children's Hospital, Harvard Medical School, Harvard School of Public Health, and the Dana Farber Cancer Institute. It showed that young leukemia patients receiving fluorinated steroids had IQs measuring a full ten points lower than those who received a nonfluorinated variety.[116]

Fluoride itself may not pose the only risk to kids' IQs. The type of fluoride compound used in about nine out of ten fluoridated communities, known as silicofluorides, may be another. In a study of 280,000 Massachusetts school children published in 1999, Dartmouth Professor Roger Masters and chemical engineer Myron Coplan reported that those from communities whose water contained silicofluorides had higher levels of lead, another substance that impairs cognitive ability.[117]

However, it's the part of the body that fluoride is supposed to benefit—the teeth—that are actually the outward indicators of the damage it causes in the form of dental fluorosis. That's a condition in which teeth initially develop white spots and streaks but eventually become discolored, brittle, and prone to breaking. It was becoming so pronounced in fluoridated locales throughout the country that in 2011, the Department of Health and Human services and the EPA jointly recommended that the amount used be lowered to 0.7 milligrams per liter (the equivalent of 0.7 parts per million).[118]

Fluoridation advocates and many dentists tend to dismiss dental fluorosis as a mere cosmetic problem. But critics of the practice claim it can have more serious implications. For example, Dr. Robert Carton, a scientist and long-time veteran of the EPA's Office of Toxic Substances, has called it "the first indication that fluoride has interfered with the enzymes in the body" where "symptoms are not visible."[119]

The greatest concern raised by the appearance of dental fluorosis is the development of an underlying and far more serious condition called skeletal fluorosis, a progressive degeneration of the bones that can lead to arthritis and hip fractures first observed in those places the ADA has referred to with high natural fluoride concentrations in their water (which, incidentally, were also the locales whose inhabitants were reported to have fewer cavities). One study, done in 2001, found that all the children exposed to excessive fluoride levels not only had dental fluorisis (with more than a third suffering serious damage to their teeth), but also that among both children and adults, a linear correlation between dental fluorosis and the frequency of bone fractures was observed.[120]

Another apparent effect of fluoride on bones is a rise in osteocarcoma, described "as a rare malignant bone tumor, commonly occurring in the age group of 10 to 24 years." First reported in a study done jointly in the 1990s by the National Cancer Institute and the New Jersey Department of Health in young males living in fluoridated parts of the state (where fluoridation is still the exception, rather than the rule), the link was recently corroborated in a 2012 study published in the *South Asian Journal of Cancer*. Noting that during periods of rapid skeleton growth fluoride uptake in bone increases, the study's authors concluded that a finding of "high serum fluoride levels in osteosarcoma patients along with high drinking water fluoride level in our patients suggest a link between fluoride and osteosarcoma."[121] (That finding, in turn, correlates with the results of tests belatedly performed by the government around 1989, which linked fluoride to excess bone cancers in young male rats.[122])

Young people aren't the only ones whose bones are apt to be adversely affected by fluoride exposure. A 1992 study published in the *Journal of the American Medical Association* found a "small but significant increase" in hip fractures in both men and women exposed to fluoridation at 1 ppm, suggesting that "low levels of fluoride may increase the risk of hip fracture in the elderly."[123]

Then there's the evidence that fluoridation may be linked to a rise in heart disease. A check of vital statistics of Grand Rapids, for example, reportedly showed that the cardiac-related death rate there nearly doubled from 585 to 1,059 in the four years following fluoridation's introduction. Additionally, after nine years of having its water fluoridated, heart disease was "responsible for a larger proportion of death in Newburgh than in most other sections of the United States," according to an editorial in the city's newspaper in January, 1954—73.9 percent higher than the national rate at that time. Indications that fluoride may damage the cardiovascular system have also been found by Japanese and Chinese researchers.[124]

Other studies, done by scientists at the International Society for Fluoride Research, have not only implicated fluoride in heart disease, but in conditions ranging from thyroid and breathing problems to arthritis to Down's syndrome.[125]

"What's extremely important to remember, another prominent fluoride researcher, now retired chemistry professor Dr. Paul Connett, once told a coauthor of this book, "is that 50 percent of the fluoride you ingest each day goes into your bones, and the level of fluoride in the bones of the American people is not being traced. From my point of view as a scientist, this represents very bad science."[126]

The scientific consensus that just isn't there

Of course, the fact that the health issues linked to fluoridation echo the concerns expressed by its original critics on the far right has made it easy for its present-day advocates to continue to label anyone who opposes it as a "crackpot," whatever their credentials. So has the support it's gotten both from lobbies such as the American Dental Association (ADA) and the US Centers for Disease Control and Prevention (CDC), which has called it one of the country's ten greatest public health achievements of the twentieth century.

But if you think such powerful backers represent some sort of scientific consensus in its favor (as they'd like you to), you'd be wrong. As it turns out, some of the strongest resistance has come from within the ranks of another government agency, one whose members are well versed in the effects of toxic agents on our health. That's the US Environmental Protection Agency (EPA). Whereas the CDC has emerged as an actual promoter of fluoridation, the EPA's role has been to regulate the levels of fluoride allowable in drinking water. As a result, some of the most outspoken critics of the practice in recent years have been top scientists from the agency, among them Dr. Carton, Dr. William L. Marcus, former senior science advisor for the EPA's drinking water program (who successfully sued over his dismissal for airing his opinions in a 1990 whistle-blowing memo about the carcinogenicity of fluoride), and Dr. William Hirzy, a former senior scientist in the Office of Pollution Prevention and Toxics.

Hirzy also served as vice president of the union that represented the toxicologists, chemists, biologists, and other professionals working at the EPA's headquarters—a union that in 1997 voted unanimously to cosponsor an initiative to reverse a California law calling for the mandatory fluoridation of certain locales. In so doing, that union, Local 2050 of the National Federation of Federal Employees, cited studies pointing to a causal link between fluoride exposure and cancer, genetic damage, bone pathology, neurological impairment, and the associated lowering of IQs in children.

"It is our hope," said a statement accompanying that endorsement, "that our cosponsorship of the Safe Drinking Water Initiative to prohibit fluoridation will have a beneficial effect on the health and welfare of all Californians by helping to keep their water free of a chemical substance for which there is substantial evidence of adverse health effects and, contrary to public perception, virtually no evidence of significant benefits.

"As the professionals who are charged with assessing the safety of drinking water, we concluded that the health and welfare of the public is not served by the addition of this substance to the public water supply," the statement concluded.[127]

However, to read the media and government hype about fluoridation, one would never suspect that its safety was anything that "real" scientists were concerned about, nor, for that matter, that its original intent was ever anything other than protecting children's teeth from cavities.

An example of this biased media coverage in favor of fluoridation is CNN's story on the federal government's recommended lowering of the amount of fluoride added to water in 2011 due to that increase in the rate of fluorosis. After stating, only four paragraphs down, that "fluoride was first added to water in the United States in the 1940s to help prevent tooth decay in children 8 years and under," it continues with what Health and Human Services Assistant Secretary for Health Dr. Howard Koh called one of its biggest advantages: "it benefits all residents of a community—at home, work, school or play," and its "effectiveness in preventing tooth decay is not limited to children, but extends throughout life, resulting in improved oral health."

The article goes on to quote ADA President Dr. Raymond F. Gist as calling the recommended reduction "a superb example of a government agency fulfilling its mission to protect and enhance the health of the American people" and applauding the HHS for "reaffirming the safety and efficacy of optimal community water fluoridation, with science on their side." It also offers an unnamed administration official's explanation for the change—that air conditioning had become more common since fluoridation began, "so children in hotter regions drank more water and needed lower levels of fluoride to protect their teeth, while children in colder climates drank less water and needed higher levels." (No, you really can't make this stuff up.)

Following all this attempted spin, however, is a statement from Jane Houlihan, senior vice president for research at the Environmental Working Group, that "the government's official, belated—and perhaps begrudging—announcement marks its recognition that fluoride policies have been out of step with the science on the tap water additive's toxicity to children, and that many American children are at risk from excess fluoride in drinking water and other sources." Such findings from the National Academy of Sciences and many others, she added, had documented "that excess fluoride exposure poses dangers that range from discolored teeth to potential hormone disruption and neurotoxicity."[128]

EPA scientists and organizations like the EWG are not the only ones to raise serious doubts about both the safety and effectiveness—as well as the morality—of a policy on which many professional reputations (such as those of CDC officials) have been staked. Fluoridation has now been officially rejected or banned in a growing list of countries, including Austria, Belgium, Germany, Finland, Denmark, Sweden, Norway, the Netherlands, Hungary, Israel, and China, home to the world's largest number of people. According to data reported by the website Fluoridation.com, 99 percent of western continental Europe had rejected, banned, or halted the practice "due to environmental, health, legal, or ethical concerns," and only five percent of the world's inhabitants were having their water fluoridated—half of whom resided in North America.[129]

The refusal of all those other countries to "get with the program" has, in turn, revealed just how hollow those claims are of the wonderful benefits of fluoridation. As Connett notes in a video compilation featured at Fluoridation.com, "The overwhelming number of countries in the world do not fluoridate—and guess what? They're teeth are just as good, if not better, than ours."[130]

That's not to mention those ethical concerns about literally forcing what fluoridation critics refer to as "mass medication" down people's throats, where it affects not just their teeth, but all their organs. (As some have pointed out, if fluoride does help strengthen enamel, it's strictly in topical applications, as in toothpaste. Even then, toothpaste containing fluoride should not be swallowed, warns the label on the box that reminds us to call a poison control center if it's ingested.)

If all this is true, then why isn't it being more widely reported? Why do well-meaning politicians continue to promote fluoridation initiatives in places where it hasn't yet been tried, claiming to have the backing of the government, scientists, and the dental profession? The answer is that fluoridation's advocates—again, many of whose reputations are on the line—have gone from stigmatizing opponents to stonewalling them.

Such refusal to even acknowledge the existence of any doubts is described by Bryson, in his book, *The Fluoride Deception*. In a section called "The Strange Case of the Missing Debaters," he offers a couple examples, including that of Tom Webster, a Boston University environmental health professor who attempted back in 2001 to initiate a debate on fluoridation, only to find that its proponents had no interest in participating.

Some were genuinely antagonistic, such as the CDC official who replied, "How dare you even hold such an event, it is really unprofessional."

When Webster finally managed to organize a discussion about the practice, he was unable to really get anyone to defend it. The topic, he noted "is just not on the radar screen. If people like Connett (who spoke at the event) are crazy, I would have loved to see the CDC people come and squash 'em like a bug. There seems to be almost a taboo about discussing this subject."[131]

Unfortunately, the health risks that continue to be caused by this ill-informed, ill-advised, and duplicitous practice have remained with us, even if its supporters think they can resolve the issue by simply not talking about it. That's why it's important that you be aware of whether or not the water supply in your community is fluoridated—and if it is, to take steps to protect yourself and your family from this insidious poison being added to both your water and your food.

Know your badditives and how to avoid them:

FLUORIDE

- If you live in a community that fluoridates its water, buy a filter that removes fluoride (not all do), such as a reverse osmosis filter. (Although this is initially more expensive than buying bottled water, it will end up saving you money in the long run.)
- Remember that any commercial products that are manufactured with water, such as juice, tea, coffee, soda, and even soup, may have been made with fluoridated water. If there's a brand you especially like, call the manufacturer to find out if it's bottled in a fluoridated location—and if so, ask if they remove the fluoride.
- Don't let your dentist surprise you with a fluoride rinse or varnish. When you're buying mouthwash and toothpaste, look for ones without added fluoride (Tom's of Maine, for instance, offers non-fluoridated toothpaste options that are sold almost everywhere.)

GMOs

The Alien Life-Forms
on Your Dinner Plate

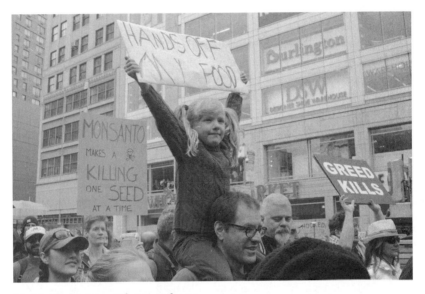

Credit: Glynnis Jones / Shutterstock.com

"In no other instance have so many scientists so seriously subverted the standards they were trained to uphold, misled so many people, and imposed such magnitude of risk on both human health and the health of the environment."
—Steven M. Druker, public interest attorney, from his book
Altered Genes, Twisted Truths

While the genetic engineering of crops is a practice that has created no small amount of controversy in recent years, the resulting genetically modified organisms, or GMOs, aren't usually thought of as food additives. Why, then, have we opted to include them in this book?

Surprisingly enough, under US law they are technically considered food additives—ones that have never been subjected to any safety testing.[132] Remember, too, that we're talking about ingredients created not by Mother Nature, but rather in a laboratory. From everything we now know about them, GMOs can be described as *badditives* for a whole bunch of reasons.

According to the corporate and government backers of crop biotechnology, GMOs, or the foods that contain them, are really just the same and every bit as safe as the conventional versions of those commodities. Except, that is, in one tiny respect: they've had a little something added on a genetic level (put there by means of either bacteria or a "gene gun") to give a crop a characteristic it wouldn't ordinarily have—like, say, being unaffected by a particular herbicide.

Such an alteration to the DNA of a living thing is actually what's known as a mutation. While that might not be a difference you can see or taste, it's apt to cause a profound change in certain characteristics of the organism in question. Then, too, the nature of the transformations that the scientists behind it consider desirable might actually be quite harmful to both human health and the environment—as we're only now belatedly starting to find out.

In that respect, what's taken place isn't all that different from the experiments depicted in those old sci-fi movies that always seemed to go awry (which is why GMOs have been given the nickname "Frankenfoods")—or, if you prefer, the classic film *Invasion of the Body Snatchers*, in which alien pods take over the bodies of everyday people whose outward appearances remain unchanged.

Just like in that movie, it's all part of an attempt to literally take over the world, or at least the world's agricultural resources, on which our very survival depends. Now, that may sound like "crazy talk"—that is, until you consider how it's designed to work, what the results have been so far, and where it may be heading unless we're armed with the knowledge and the determination to protect ourselves and to reverse the course of events before it's too late.

The unforeseen consequences of messing with Mother Nature's building blocks

Before we even go into the bizarre background story of how GMOs were allowed to invade our farmlands and food supply (a subject on which much has been written), there's something you need to know right up front. It's the fact that whatever you may have heard about how completely "safe" genetically modified foods are, and how they're essentially no different from those that haven't been bioengineered, it is all part of an elaborate con job—one designed to protect the profits of both Big Food and the biotechnology industry at the expense of your family's health.

Perhaps the best indicator of how patently false those notions are comes from those consumers whose honesty you can always depend on—the animals in our midst. As Jeffrey M. Smith, executive director of the Institute for Responsible Technology, notes in his book, *Genetic Roulette*, when given the choice, animals usually make a point of steering clear of genetically altered foods.

- Geese that landed annually on an Illinois pond and habitually fed on an adjacent fifty-acre soybean field wouldn't go near the Roundup Ready GM soybeans newly planted on half of the field, according to agricultural writer C. F. Marley. They continued to eat the conventional soybeans on the other side.
- Cows in Iowa refused to eat from a trough containing genetically modified (GM) Bt corn, opting for one containing corn that hadn't been genetically engineered instead.
- Some cattle ignored a field of Roundup Ready corn and actually broke through a fence to get to a field of non-GM corn.[133]

Are they merely being finicky, or might those geese, cows, and other creatures who have exhibited similar reactions know something we don't? It certainly seems that way, given what researchers have discovered about the effects of GMOs on animals in studies that have been conducted. After ingesting Roundup Ready soy, the livers and testicular cells in mice underwent changes and their pancreases stopped functioning normally. The offspring of mother rats fed the same type of soy died at more than five times the rate of those whose mothers were given a nonbioengineered variety. That's not to mention the sheep and cows that reportedly died after feeding on genetically engineered Bt cotton and corn.[134]

It turns out there's an awful lot we don't know about the hidden effects of altering an organism's DNA, and the consequences on any person or creature that happens to consume it.

Despite the lack of any official safety testing on GMOs (more on that in a moment), the evidence that has accumulated so far has been sufficient to suggest that transferring genes from one life–form to another can have unanticipated and unintended biological consequences.

Such genetic engineering "can change the metabolism of a plant or animal," according to Martha Herbert, a pediatric neurologist and neuroscientist at Massachusetts General Hospital. "Proteins may be produced in increased quantities. Proteins that in small quantities were safe may now even exceed toxic levels. New proteins may be produced that were not produced before." And that can lead to "changes in function, or changes in potential for allergy."[135]

Perhaps that accounts for why soy allergies among 4,500 people tested in the United Kingdom rose from 10 to 15 percent just after Roundup Ready soy began to be imported (Monsanto's own study, in fact, found it contained 27 percent more of a known allergen than non-GM soy). Given that soybean proteins can also trigger reactions to peanuts, it also might explain why peanut allergies doubled among children in the United States during the five-year period after GM soy was first marketed here.[136]

It's certainly a plausible explanation for the symptoms suffered by about one hundred people living near a Bt cornfield in the Philippines, who experienced "headaches, dizziness, extreme stomach pains, fever, and allergies" after inhaling pollen that was shed by the corn, with thirty-nine who were tested showing a Bt toxin antibody response.[137] Or for a supposedly harmless pest-resistant protein in beans causing airway inflammation and allergic lung damage in mice when transferred to peas by Australian researchers, who were forced to abandon the experiment.[138]

In fact, the potential of a protein gone awry may be even worse than an allergic reaction. For example, according to cell biologist Barry Commoner, the protein could conceivably become misshapen or misfolded in the absence of what he calls a "chaperone" protein in its natural environment. While that might deactivate it in some cases, in others it might have a pernicious effect, Mad Cow Disease being an example of what can happen when a misfolded protein replicates itself in the brain.[139]

Glyphosate—the other half of the GMO "hidden hazard" equation

The unforeseen consequences of tampering with Mother Nature's biological building blocks are not the only area of concern many experts have about so many of our basic foods that have become genetically engineered. There's also the chief purpose such DNA remodeling serves, which is to make the resulting crops "Roundup Ready"—that is, to be able to survive being doused with Monsanto's Roundup, currently the world's most widely used herbicide, whose main ingredient, glyphosate, was declared a probable cause of cancer by the International Agency for Research on Cancer (IARC), a World Health Organization subsidiary, in 2015.

Even before IARC announced that finding, research on the health effects of glyphosate suggested it may be linked to a number of other serious illnesses. A 2013 article in the scientific journal *Entropy* pointed out that the chemical can interfere with the biochemistry of beneficial bacteria that humans depend on to synthesize essential amino acids, and that prolonged consumption may therefore predispose humans to a host of chronic health problems, ranging from obesity and depression to autism, inflammatory bowel disease, Alzheimer's, and Parkinson's.[140]

Unfortunately, glyphosate is everywhere these days. As Agricultural Economist Charles Benbrook, PhD, has observed, "no pesticide has come remotely close to such intensive and widespread use" in the United States. According to a paper published by Benbrook in February 2016 in the peer-reviewed journal *Environmental Sciences Europe*, the global use of glyphosate has risen almost fifteen-fold since Roundup Ready crops were introduced in 1996 with two-thirds of the total amount applied in the US from 1974 to 2014 having been sprayed in just the last ten years of that period.[141]

Unlike other agricultural chemicals, however, no one was even attempting to monitor the amounts of glyphosate being harbored in foods, until early in 2016 when the FDA finally announced plans to conduct such testing.

What took them so long? According to a spokesperson, more "streamlined" methods of detection had been developed to replace the "very cost- and labor-intensive" ones previously available.[142] A sneak preview of what the results might be was provided by Norwegian researchers in 2014, who reported finding high residues of glyphosate in bioengineered soybeans, but none in either non-GMO or organic soy, leading them to suggest that lack of data on such residues in major crops "is a serious gap of knowledge with potential consequences for human and animal health."[143]

How a judicial and political coupling gave birth to today's GMOs

As with other devious schemes, ranging from prison breaks to big-time jewel heists, the unleashing of GMOs on an unsuspecting public could not have been accomplished without a considerable amount of "inside help" from the very people whose job it was to keep such breaches from taking place.

It all started with a US Supreme Court decision that allowed certain life-forms to be considered private property.

That came about back in 1980, when the high court ruled in a 5–4 decision that a scientist named Ananda Chakrabarty could own the intellectual property rights to a genetically engineered oil-eating bacterium after the US Patent and Trademark Office initially denied the claim on the grounds that living things "are not patentable subject matter." While the majority agreed that laws of nature, physical phenomena, and abstract ideas could not be patented, they contended that genetically engineered organisms were "manufactured," rather than a product of nature, and therefore covered by patent law. It also noted that patents were intended to protect "unforeseen advances."[144,145]

Just how "unforeseen" the consequences of that decision would be, however, would become all too apparent in the advances that followed.

While the first biotech application to pass muster with the FDA came in 1982 in the form of a synthetic form of insulin produced by genetically modified bacteria, it would take another decade for the FDA to put its stamp of approval on the marketing of GMOs for food use.

The FDA official who was most responsible for that was none other than Michael Taylor, a former attorney for the Monsanto Corp. of St. Louis (which in the late 1990s had divested itself of its longtime—and often controversial—chemical business to become a firm specializing in agricultural products). But Taylor didn't magically materialize on the regulatory scene. Like the appointment of Arthur Hull Hayes, the FDA commissioner who approved the neurotoxic sweetener NutraSweet (the patented version of aspartame, later bought by Monsanto), his arrival was actually the result of a politico-economic policy, one that also began during Ronald Reagan's presidency.

The first indication of this was the development of "a Coordinated Framework for the Regulation of Biotechnology to provide for the regulatory oversight of organisms derived through genetic engineering" by the federal government in 1986.[146] The following year, according to an account featured in the *Huffington Post* Green blog *Green*, "then-Vice President George H. W. Bush visited a Monsanto lab for a photo op with the developers of Roundup Ready crops. According to a video report of the meeting, when Monsanto executives worried about the approval process for their new crops, Bush laughed and told them, 'Call me. We're in the dereg business. Maybe we can help.'"[147]

Help he did, when five years later, as Reagan's successor, he assigned his own veep, Dan Quayle, to get a "regulatory relief initiative" for GMO crops underway. At a press conference, Quayle, who headed what was known as the "Competitiveness Council," touted biotech's potential profitability "as long as we resist the spread of unnecessary regulations." One way to do that was for the administration to appoint Taylor, who proceeded to have genetically engineered crops declared "the substantial equivalent" of conventional ones, therefore requiring neither safety testing nor special labeling[148]—a regulatory paradox, given that the same GMOs were considered to be substantially different enough to merit an actual patent. (It's also a claim that, at least in the case of soybeans, was contradicted by that aforementioned Norwegian study, which concluded that, based on thirty-five different variables, "without exception" there was "substantial non-equivalence" between the three different types of ready-to-market soybeans.[149])

All this was accomplished with very little general awareness of what was occurring at the time—as well as of its implications for food production. It did, however, arouse the attention of Steven M. Druker, a public interest attorney who ended up initiating legal action to have this FDA policy reversed. While that litigation ultimately was deflected, it did give Druker access to the innermost details of what had taken place in the form of 44,000 pages of documents, which he came to regard as "extensive evidence of an enormous, ongoing fraud," one involving evasion of both laws and scientific standards that, as he recounted in his 2015 book, *Altered Genes, Twisted Truths*, had subjected the American people to "novel foods that were abnormally risky in the eyes of the agency's own scientists."[150]

Druker did not come to that conclusion based on a paper trail alone. He also relied on sources with an inside knowledge of how GMOs came to be accepted with no safety testing, a major one being the biologist Philip Regal, who revealed to him how the interests of investors in the success of the new technology resulted in customary scientific caution being thrown to the winds. Contrary to initial assurances he had received, Regal told him, the attitude he heard expressed at a 1988 conference on the subject by both industry and government officials was, "if the American people want progress, they are going to have to be the guinea pigs."[151]

That same term, as Druker notes further on, was used a decade later by another scientist, renowned food safety expert Arpad Pusztai, a veteran of the prestigious Rowett Research Institute in Aberdeen, Scotland, who had been chosen by the Scottish Agriculture, Environment and Fisheries Department to verify the safety of genetically engineered food. After an extensive study of a pesticide-producing potato developed by Monsanto and its effects on lab rats, however, Pusztai, with the permission of the Institute's director, expressed concerns about the safety of GMOs to a British TV interviewer, saying he found it "very, very unfair to use our fellow citizens as guinea pigs. We have to find the guinea pigs in the laboratory."

Two day later, the scientist was not only fired, but his project was terminated and his data confiscated, reportedly at the behest of Prime Minister Tony Blair (according to a 2003 article in the *Daily Mail*) following a phone call from then-President Bill Clinton, another big proponent of biotechnology. This account was substantiated by two other researchers at Rowett.[152]

The stranglehold on seeds

The stage was now set for Monsanto's takeover of America's farm land and food supply—one it would also attempt in other parts of the world, only with substantially more resistance and less success than in the US.

The opening act of this unprecedented power play was actually one that ended up being yanked off the stage. Not because it was tasteless, as critics claimed, nor because even lab rats rejected it and had to be force-fed it via gastric tubes, nor because a number of them developed stomach lesions and seven of forty died within two weeks of eating one variety.[153] No, the FlavrSavr Tomato, which was designed to be firmer and to last longer through the genetic inhibition of a natural protein, simply wasn't the profitable production number its creators had hoped it would be. So Monsanto, which bought out the firm that developed it, simply ended its run.

The company actually had plans for biotech that were far more grandiose, an elaborate scheme that involved both taking control of the seeds for major food crops and using them as a means of skyrocketing the sales of its glyphosate-based weed killer, Roundup. In only a few short years, with the cooperation of not just the FDA but also the US Department of Agriculture, it had managed to do just that. Within the next couple decades, it had not only developed and patented Roundup Ready® seeds for a whole bevy of commodities, but also managed to convince the great majority of US growers to switch over to them with promises of a weed-free future. As a result, by 2014, over 90 percent of the country's field corn, soybean, canola, cotton (the source of cottonseed oil), and sugar beet acreage had been genetically modified, mostly for the purpose of accommodating Roundup, in addition to smaller percentages of the alfalfa fed to farm animals and, most recently, sweet corn (the kind you eat on the cob).[154]

Monsanto has also for some time been incorporating into its Roundup Ready corn varieties the insect-killing toxin found in Bt corn, its initial entry in the GMO field, which comes from the soil bacterium *Bacillus thuringiensis,* according to Bill Freese, science policy analyst for the nonprofit Center for Food Safety.[155]

Monsanto, of course, would like us to think that the popularity of its Roundup Ready seeds must be deserved. However, what it doesn't mention are the strategies it has devised to dominate the marketplace with both its seeds and its herbicide—for example, engineering the seeds so that those purchasing them had no choice but to use Roundup on the resultant crops after its patent had expired,[156] as well as gradually buying up heirloom and conventional seed enterprises. As Freese has pointed out, "high-quality conventional seeds are rapidly disappearing, thanks to the biotech multinationals' tightening stranglehold on the world's seed supply."[157]

There's also the fact that customers for Monsanto's transgenic seeds aren't allowed to save them for the next planting, as has traditionally been the practice in farming. Instead, they're obligated to buy new ones from the company every year in accordance with their purchasing agreement. Those who have violated that contract have found themselves taken to court by Monsanto for patent infringement, to the tune of an estimated $85 million in court-imposed and pretrial settlements by 2009.[158]

Such "seed servitude," as Freese calls it, isn't the only unanticipated drawback this arrangement has had for many farmers. There's also been the widespread appearance of Roundup-resistant "superweeds," just the sort of counterproductive effect that pesticide dependency inevitably brings about. (However, that problem, they've been told, should finally be resolved, at least for now, through the application of a significantly stronger herbicide, Dow's Enlist Duo, a combination of glyphosate and 2,4-D, given final approval by the Environmental Protection Agency in 2016, with corresponding seeds to follow).

The problems caused by so much of our farmland being given over to transgenic crops go beyond those faced by the farmers who plant them, however. Also threatened with potential litigation are noncustomers, whose fields are often contaminated by wind-blown Monsanto seeds, which are even a threat to organic agriculture.

GMO labeling: the homefront battle that's already been won abroad

The near monopoly that Monsanto, in just a few short years, has mana-ged to gain in this manner over some of our most basic agricultural com-modities is reflected on supermarket shelves, where well over 80 percent of processed foods now contain genetically modified ingredients. While the powers that be have been fully cooperative in allowing that take-over to take place, the same can't be said for the buying public, many of whom, despite the safety assurances of both government and industry representatives, have formed what amounts to a full-scale resistance movement.

For one thing, they've been demanding something now required in five dozen other countries—the labeling of GMOs. Such labeling was, in fact, required under a Vermont law that took effect in July 2016, only to be superseded by a bipartisan bill passed by Congress and signed by President Obama at the end of that month, which required GMO labeling only on Smartphone apps, rather than on actual labels. This revised "compromise" version of what came to be known as "the DARK Act" (for Deny Americans the Right to Know), also calls for a study by the USDA to determine whether enough consumers have "access to electronic disclosures," with "alternative methods of disclosure" to be provided if they're found not to. Even without such clear and straightforward labeling, a substantial number of shoppers have limited their buying habits either to certified organic foods, in which GMOs are expressly prohibited, or to products bearing the seal of the Non-GMO Project, which tests all ingredients that could be genetically modified prior to approving any item.

The rebellion even had its own contemporary version of the Boston Tea Party, with the deliberate destruction of 6,500 acres of Roundup Ready sugar beets in Oregon during two nights in June 2013, an act condemned as both criminal and cowardly by the state's top agricultural official, "regardless of how one feels about biotechnology"[159]—but one that appears to have been a form of protest against the 'mutation without representation' those GMOs symbolized.

Such pressure from the public, to be sure, has brought results—most notably agreements from some mainstream food companies, such as Campbell's Soup, General Mills, and Mars, to begin labeling products containing GMOs, as well as a pledge from the Chipotle restaurant chain to simply stop using genetically modified ingredients.

Despite such concessions, however, and recent surveys that have found that more than 90 percent of Americans are in favor of GMO labeling, forces in both industry and government have gone to considerable lengths in their efforts to convince consumers that their concerns are unfounded.

One of the latest such efforts was a report released in May 2016 by the National Academy of Sciences that purported to have found "no evidence" that GMOs were unsafe to eat or had adverse environmental impacts, and which saw no need for their being labeled.[160] However, as was quickly pointed out by the consumer advocacy group Food & Water Watch, the Academy's research arm, the National Research Council (NRC), has strong ties to industry that "have created conflicts of interest at every level," having taken millions of dollars in funding from biotechnology companies and invited sponsors like Monsanto to sit on high-level boards overseeing its work.[161]

The report is also most revealing in what it acknowledges—that these industry-affiliated scientists were unable to come up with any evidence that genetically modified crops have increased potential yields, supposedly the main rationale for having allowed these alien organisms to invade the agricultural scene in the first place. (In other words, they won't succeed in "feeding the world.")

While GMO labeling would certainly be an important step in advancing the ability of consumers to avoid products containing mutant ingredients, Steven Druker has reservations about how effective it would be and whether it could withstand a court challenge. In his opinion, what we need is nothing less than a complete prohibition on and phase-out of genetically engineered crops, based on having to prove a substance is GRAS (generally recognized as safe) through "rigorous safety testing" before it can be marketed, as is already required by existing law. While acknowledging that this would involve significant complications, he contends it is "far better to weather whatever short-term economic difficulties may be entailed than to suffer the long-term health and environmental damage that could result from inaction."[162]

Of course, whether any president, public official, or jurist would be forward-thinking and bold enough to order such a belated ban remains to be seen. The food industry itself well might, however, if only citizens were to "exert their collective influence," as he puts it.[163] And that's where labeling could play an important role.

For while Monsanto and its biotech allies may be able to use their considerable clout, resources, and influence to buy or intimidate scientists and coerce farmers, lawmakers, and bureaucrats (as they've been doing for years), there's one force they can't control, and that's the power of informed consumers.

Once enough members of the public refuse to be used any longer as guinea pigs by simply saying "no" to the risky and unnatural fruits of this ill-conceived experiment, the companies that have been its enablers will have no choice but to reverse course—and we can begin to reclaim our food supply from these mutant life-forms and their corporate creators.

How Monsanto's seed-leasing contract stymies safety research on GMOs

Is "freedom of information" on the safety aspects of GMOs being deliberately blocked by the same seed-leasing agreement with Monsanto that prevents farmers from saving its genetically engineered seeds from one planting season to another?

Apparently so, according to agricultural and biotech consultant Martha Crouch, PhD, who has pointed out that the contract includes a specific prohibition on transferring such seeds to anyone else "for crop breeding, research or generation of herbicide registration data"—something she herself discovered when asked by a colleague if she could provide him with some Roundup Ready seeds for glyphosate research.

In an essay originally published in 2013 and reprinted in the book, *The GMO Deception*, Crouch notes that this stipulation is one that allows the companies whose profits might be affected by such research to determine who is and isn't allowed to conduct it.

The result, she asserts, has often been to nip research efforts by graduate students in the bud, or hinder those that seem to be going in an unfavorable direction. And while "some scientists rise to the challenge," her sense is that "many more find it too much of a hassle and decide to work on other issues."

Had she been able to obtain the seeds at issue for her friend, Crouch added, "we would know about glyphosate levels in pollen and nectar by now, and thus be better equipped to assess environmental impacts."[164]

Know your badditives and how to avoid them:

GMOs

- Without any easy-to-understand federal labeling mandate, the only sure way to avoid GMO ingredients is to stick with organic processed foods, or ones that have the Non-GMO Project verified label on the packaging.
- Avoid any product containing nonorganic soy, corn, and canola, which are most likely to be genetically modified.
- Look for products that contain "cane sugar." Foods and beverages that just say "sugar" on the ingredient label are likely to contain GM beet sugar.
- Be aware that certain types of produce may now be genetically engineered as well, including papayas, squash, and sweet corn (which has been made available to farmers but is apparently not all that popular).
- Avoid foods that contain cottonseed oil—something you'll now find in a lot of nut products. Remember, 90 percent of US cotton crops are now genetically modified.

HIGH FRUCTOSE CORN SYRUP

It Does a Body Bad

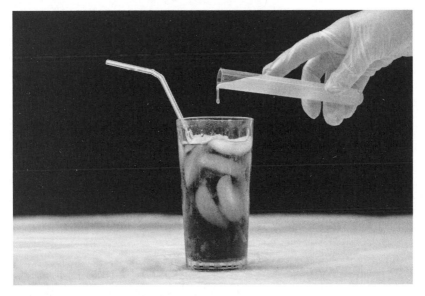

Credit: Ryan Morrill Photography

"I will predict to you that high fructose corn syrup is going to turn out to be one of the very worst culprits in the diet—a direct driver of obesity in kids, and one of the single worst things you can give to people that have the genetic constitution that predisposes them to insulin resistance, which is the basis of type 2 diabetes and a lot of the obesity that we see in the country today."
    —Andrew Weil, MD, author, nutrition, and wellness expert

High fructose corn syrup, or HFCS, first began showing up as a food and beverage ingredient more than three decades ago for reasons that had nothing to do with health—and everything to do with food industry profits.

As cane sugar prices began rising, largely due to quotas and tariffs, the cost of government-subsidized corn started falling. This just happened to coincide with a strange new sweetener, one much cheaper than sugar, that was then becoming available.

The sweetener was the sort of concoction that could have come out of a mad scientist's laboratory. Manufacturing it is a complicated process involving an enzyme called glucose isomerase, developed back in 1957, which can magically turn the glucose in corn into fructose.

The resulting gooey, syrupy white substance is really, really sweet—so sweet that, in 1984, the soft drink world's big brothers, Coke and Pepsi, began using it to replace sugar in their beverages. Before long, it had begun appearing in just about every type of processed food and drink imaginable, from yogurt, soup, and ketchup to bread, peanut butter, and jelly.

Of course, like so many other things added or done to our food for economic reasons, no one really bothered to figure out if consuming all that high fructose corn syrup might be having any sort of adverse effect on the health of consumers—at least, not initially. However, as we've since discovered to our dismay, HFCS is sickeningly sweet—a major factor in the rapid rise of a whole slew of health problems now plaguing us, ranging from obesity diabetes to fatty liver disease and pancreatic cancer. It may even be an impediment to those recovering from traumatic brain injuries.

While the corn refining industry has done its best to try to convince us that their product has been unfairly blamed for the skyrocketing increase in such infirmities, independent scientific research has increasingly confirmed that their relationship to the ubiquitous use of HFCS is anything but purely coincidental.

The "sugar coating" of an artificial laboratory sweetener

Anyone familiar with the classic film *Gone with the Wind* will remember the put-down that Scarlett O'Hara gives to her second husband, Frank Kennedy, whom she has married for money rather than love:

"Don't call me sugar!"

Well, if high fructose corn syrup could talk, it might say the same thing.

The fact is that this ultra-cheap, government-subsidized artificial sweetener (yes, that's what it actually is) has been "sugar coated" for far too long. That's especially true in regard to its use in sodas, which are commonly referred to as "sugary drinks" or "sugar-sweetened beverages," when, in reality, they contain not an iota of actual sugar (otherwise known as sucrose). "The universal sweetener in our country has become high fructose corn syrup," renowned nutrition expert Dr. Andrew Weil has pointed out, adding: "It's very hard to find things made with sugar."[165]

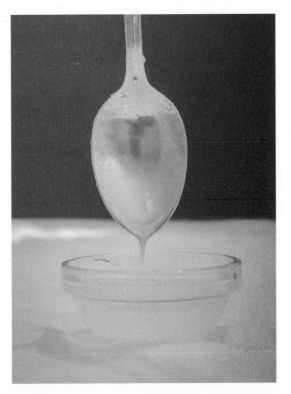

This is actual high fructose corn syrup, which bears no resemblance to the honey-like substance depicted in Internet images. *Credit: Ryan Morrill Photography*

So, why the deliberate misidentification of HFCS? It's a question we've occasionally asked of supposed experts who should know better than to use such misleading language when talking about research in which they're involved. From their responses, we can only gather that *sugar* and *sugary* have become a kind of shorthand that's much less complicated to use for descriptive purposes than talking about a sweetener created in a laboratory to substitute for actual sugar.

But is it meaningful to us as consumers whether the ingredient in question is called *sugar* or HFCS? Not according to the corn-refining industry, and those who echo its rhetoric. They've been trying to tell us for years that there's no essential difference between these sweetening agents, or how differently they affect us, and so it shouldn't really matter how we refer to them.

The Corn Refiners Association (CRA), for instance, has long asserted that "in terms of composition, high fructose corn syrup is nearly identical to table sugar (sucrose), which is composed of 50 percent fructose and 50 percent glucose."[166] It even petitioned the Food and Drug Administration to allow "high fructose corn syrup" to have its name officially changed to "corn sugar," a proposed name it promoted in an ad campaign called "Sweet Surprise."

However, the FDA refused to go along with that request. One reason was because it defines sugar as "a solid, dried, and crystallized food; whereas syrup is an aqueous solution or liquid food." The other reason was that "corn sugar" was already the official name for dextrose (which contains no fructose, only glucose). Additionally, calling HFCS by the same name as a product that's fructose-free would be highly confusing to people who needed to avoid fructose for medical reasons.

Coming from the FDA, that was quite a rebuke, especially given that agency's long record of leniency toward the processed food industry's requests. But it didn't stop the CRA from continuing to maintain that HFCS was "a form of sugar and nutritionally the same as other sugars." What makes this claim all the more confusing is the fact that the FDA uses the term "sugars" as a synonym for all caloric sweeteners.

In addition to the fact that HFCS is clearly not the same thing as sugar, neither are all so-called "sugars" the same in terms of their effects on health. Some natural sugars, such as maple syrup and honey, have been shown to have various nutritional and biological benefits.

As "sugars" go, however, what researchers have discovered about HFCS, combined with what has occurred during its relatively brief history, should be enough to make us want to avoid it whenever and wherever possible.

And don't confuse HFCS with corn syrup, either

It's a media misnomer you see quite often in news stories and particularly in headlines—a reference to corn syrup, when the story is really about high fructose corn syrup.

In reality, HFCS is no more corn syrup than it is corn sugar.

Corn syrup (which, unlike HFCS, is readily available in food stores), is a product that's been used for decades by everyday cooks in recipes such as pecan pie. It's also 100 percent glucose, which means it contains no fructose whatsoever. So, while your grandma may well have used corn syrup, unless she was a chemist, she never would have used high fructose corn syrup.

Unfortunately, the thing today's corn syrup does have in common with HFCS is that both are likely made from genetically modified corn. The health hazards posed by GMOs, which also include beet sugar as opposed to cane sugar, is a subject also discussed in this book.

However, let there be no mistake: HFCS is neither sugar, corn sugar, nor corn syrup, despite anything you may read to the contrary.

The HFCS–obesity connection

Let's begin with one of the key differences between cane sugar, long used to sweeten products ranging from soda to relish, and HFCS, which has replaced it in most of these items—the fact that the latter is much more apt to make you fat.

Now, the Corn Refiners Association would like you to believe the idea that HFCS is a "unique contributor" to obesity is a "myth" with "no scientific evidence" to back it up and that weight gain is merely caused "by consuming more calories than are expended."[167] But that first claim has been disproven time and time again as plenty of evidence has been produced by researchers showing a clear biological link between HFCS consumption and obesity. The second one ignores the fact that all calories are not created equal, any more than all sugars are.

One thing we know for sure: in the last few decades, the American public has put on a tremendous amount of weight. In fact, more than a third of us are now considered obese, in contrast to 1970, when the number was approximately half of that. While this might seem like a normal state of affairs to people in their teens or twenties, it's dramatically different from the world those of us who grew up in the 1950s, '60s, or even '70s can recall.

Can the addition of HFCS to our diet be blamed for this huge change in our physical makeup? After all, it's well recognized that technology has been largely responsible for making us a far more sedentary society. Is a change in lifestyle all that's behind it, as the corn refining industry would have us think?

Perhaps not. One thing even the CRA can't deny is that the fattening up of America seems to have corresponded with the infusion of HFCS into all manner of processed foods, including many we might not ordinarily think of as needing sweetening, such as mayonnaise and bread (making for a double whammy in that sandwich!)

Of course, part of the explanation for this is the fact that HFCS has replaced sugar in nearly all soft drinks—and because it's so much cheaper than cane sugar, the typical bottle or serving of soda has gotten much bigger (compared to some other products that have actually been downsized). Additionally, as scientists have discovered, there appears to be a lot more at work in the way HFCS packs on the pounds.

One study that attested to this phenomenon was conducted by Princeton researchers back in 2010. They found that rats given HFCS gained significantly more weight than those fed table sugar, despite the fact that both groups consumed roughly the same number of calories.

As was noted by professor Bart Hoebel, a specialist in appetite, weight, and sugar addiction, every single participating rat "across the board" became obese when "drinking high-fructose corn syrup at levels well below those in soda pop," something not even seen in those fed a high-fat diet. "Some people have claimed that high-fructose corn syrup is no different than other sweeteners when it comes to weight gain and obesity," he added, "but our results make it clear that this just isn't true, at least under the conditions of our tests."[168]

That's not all. As graduate student Miriam Bocarsly observed, "These rats aren't just getting fat; they're demonstrating characteristics of obesity, including substantial increases in abdominal fat and circulating triglycerides. In humans, these same characteristics are known risk factors for high blood pressure, coronary artery disease, cancer and diabetes."[169] (More on that in a moment.)

In fact, those results were based on all calories being equal. That's something that's not likely to happen with the consumption of HFCS, according to a Canadian rat study done in 2013, which found that the higher the doses of HFCS the animals were given, the more they wanted and the harder they worked to get it. By comparison, rats given similar amounts of saccharine, whose initial response was the same, soon "had enough."

"The [rats'] intake of the fructose is very much related to its concentration," said Dr. Francesco Leri, an associate professor of neuroscience and applied cognitive science at the University of Guelph in Ontario. "When you change the percentage of the solution, the behavior changes, and the most compelling and most interesting evidence we have is that as you increase the percentage [of HFCS], the animals work harder and harder for each infusion."[170]

This response, Leri claimed, is "the same type of pattern" found in drug abuse. It's also similar to what was found in a University of Southern California study of twenty human volunteers whose brain blood flow, when tracked with MRI scans, showed that when they were given excessive fructose, their feeling of having "had enough" was suppressed.

Is the fructose in HFCS really all that excessive? The CRA says it's really not that much different from the amount in table sugar, either 42 or 55 percent as compared to 50 percent in sucrose. That 55 percent, however, is actually 10 percent more than the level in sugar, with some studies showing soft drinks containing levels up to 20 percent higher than that.

However, that's not the only misrepresentation of the actual amount of fructose people may be consuming in processed foods. As we discovered in the course of writing the blog Food Identity Theft for Citizens for Health, a General Mills cereal that claimed to contain "no high fructose corn syrup" listed "fructose" among its ingredients. That, according to a CRA website, is actually another name for HFCS-90, which is 90 percent fructose and "sometimes used in natural and 'light' foods, where very little is needed to provide sweetness." It continues to note: "Syrups with 90% fructose will not state high fructose corn syrup on the label, they will state 'fructose' or 'fructose syrup.'"[171]

There's something else the corn refining industry fails to mention: the fructose molecules in sugar are bound together with the glucose molecules, whereas those in HFCS are not, allowing them to be far more readily absorbed. All that may play a significant role in making HFCS a far more fattening sweetener than the sugar to which it's supposedly equivalent.

To make things worse, obesity isn't the only HFCS-related health problem for which there's plenty of scientific evidence.

Connecting the dots to diabetes

Like its refusal to acknowledge a link between HFCS and obesity, the corn-refining industry has also consistently engaged in diabetes denial, which is to say any connection between the sudden upsurge in type 2 diabetes and its laboratory-formulated sweetener.

According to recent statistics, the incidence of type 2 diabetes among children and adolescents has "skyrocketed" from less than 5 percent in 1994 to about 20 percent of all newly diagnosed cases—what the journal *Diabetes Care* has referred to as an "emerging epidemic." Not very long ago type 2 diabetes was practically unheard of in people under the age of thirty.

In fact, the number of kids with diabetes has become so immense that there's now a support group called Students with Diabetes with chapters on several dozen college campuses, including a number of state universities. Only a few decades ago, that would have been unimaginable. Except for those with type 1, or "juvenile diabetes," this was simply not a disease that affected young people until quite recently.

How did this happen? Well, consider what some very reputable research facilities have discovered in recent years about the relationship between HFCS consumption and type 2 diabetes (and these are just a couple examples):

- In 2012, a joint study conducted by the University of Southern California and Britain's University of Oxford found that countries whose food supplies contained HFCS had a 20 percent higher rate of diabetes than those where it wasn't used. The research, published in the journal *Global Public Health*, also found that this "significantly increased prevalence of diabetes" was unrelated to either total sugar consumption or obesity levels in the 42 countries examined.

Those results, said Professor Michael Goran, director of the Childhood Obesity Research Center and codirector of the Diabetes and Obesity Research Institute at the Keck School of Medicine at USC, added to "a growing body of scientific literature" showing that "HFCS consumption may result in negative health consequences distinct from and more deleterious than natural sugar." They also prompted him to note that "HFCS appears to pose a serious public health problem on a global scale."[172]

- A 2007 Rutgers University study uncovered evidence that HFCS-sweetened soft drinks contributed to the development of diabetes, particularly in children. Chemical tests of eleven different carbonated beverages containing HFCS found what the lead researcher called "astonishingly high" levels of reactive carbonyls associated with unbound fructose and glucose molecules, which do just the sort of damage that can result in the disease. By contrast, no such reactive carbonyls are present in table sugar, the fructose and glucose components of which are "bound" and thus chemically stable, he pointed out.[173]

If that's not enough to convince you why anything containing HFCS is unfit for human consumption, hang on! The ways it does a body bad get even worse.

Look out, liver, pancreas, heart, brain—here it comes!

HFCS, as it turns out, isn't just an ingredient that's apt to make you fat and diabetic; it's also a kind of equal opportunity destroyer of your vital organs. Here's just some of what researchers have discovered in recent years about the effects of consuming this supposedly benign substance:

- Unlike the natural fructose bound together with fiber in fruit, HFCS, in the words of Dr. Al Sears, a board-certified clinical nutrition specialist, "floods your bloodstream, overwhelming your liver's processing capacity."[174] Perhaps that's why a 2008 study done by the University of Florida Division of Nephrology found that patients with nonalcoholic fatty liver disease (NAFLD) consumed two to three times more fructose than controls, leading researchers to conclude that development of the disease may be associated with excessive dietary fructose.[175] Another study from Duke University Medical Center in 2010 resulted in a finding that HFCS consumption is linked to liver scarring in NAFLD patients.[176]

To put that research in perspective, NAFLD, which can often accompany both obesity and diabetes, is a condition that causes the liver to accumulate fat resembling that found in the livers of alcoholics. About 10 percent of patients will develop a much more serious form that can lead to life-threatening problems like cirrhosis of the liver, liver cancer, and liver failure.

Here's the kicker: NAFLD, which wasn't discovered until the 1980s (around the time HFCS use became widespread), is now becoming epidemic. In fact, Dr. John Helzberg, the lead researcher for that Saint Luke's study, noted that "if current trends continue, the prevalence of NAFLD is expected to increase to 40 percent of the population by 2020."[177]

- In 2010, a team of UCLA cancer researchers concluded that pancreatic cancers use fructose to activate a key cellular pathway that drives cell division, helping the cancer to grow more quickly and that "cancer cells can readily metabolize fructose to increase proliferation."
- A 2011 Georgia Health Sciences University study of 559 adolescents aged fourteen to eighteen, who consume more fructose than any other age group, found such higher fructose consumption to be associated with multiple markers of cardiometabolic risk.[178]
- Another study, led by Kimber Stanhope of the University of California at Davis, examined 48 adults between ages eighteen and forty and found that those who consumed HFCS for two weeks as 25 percent of their daily calorie requirement had increased blood levels of cholesterol and triglycerides, which are considered indicators of increased risk for heart disease.[179]

Finally, there's what can happen to "your brain on HFCS," as shown by some alarming recent findings. A 2012 UCLA peer-reviewed rat study revealed how regular consumption of fructose-laden food slows the functioning of the brain. As Fernando Gomez-Pinilla, a professor of neurosurgery, observed, "Eating a high-fructose diet over the long term alters your brain's ability to learn and remember information." (The researchers also found that a diet high in omega-3 fatty acids can help offset that disruption.)[180]

That isn't all those UCLA neuroscientists have discovered about the havoc HFCS can wreak inside your head. Another rat study they reported on in 2015 led them to conclude that it can also hinder an individual's ability to recover from traumatic brain injury. "We found that processed fructose (the kind found in HFCS, not fruit) inflicts surprisingly harmful effects on the brain's ability to repair itself after a head trauma," said Gomez-Pinilla of the team's latest research. "Our findings suggest that fructose disrupts plasticity—the creation of fresh pathways between brain cells that occurs when we learn or experience something new." He added, "That's a huge obstacle for anyone to overcome—but especially for a TBI patient, who is often struggling to relearn daily routines and how to care for himself or herself."[181]

And lest we forget the lungs . . .

Might the prevalence of HFCS in the food supply also be contributing to a sharp rise in childhood asthma rates over the past three decades? It's a distinct possibility, given the results of some recent research, including:

- A 2013 CDC study of nearly 16,000 high school students, which found that drinking three or more sodas a day increased the incidence of asthma by 64 percent, and two a day increased the risk by 28 percent.[182]
- A study of 1,100 mothers, both during and after pregnancy, supported by the National Institutes of Health and reported on at the 2015 meeting of the American Academy of Allergy, Asthma and Immunology, which showed that the likelihood of developing asthma in midchildhood rose by 22 percent for kids whose mothers consumed large quantities of fructose during the second trimester of pregnancy.[183]

If that's not bad enough, another 2015 study of more than 2,800 adults between ages twenty and fifty-five, done by researchers from the New York Medical College and the University of Massachusetts, found that drinking five or more sodas containing HFCS per week increased the incidence of chronic bronchitis by more than 80 percent![184]

All of these are more reasons why we might literally be able to breathe easier once HFCS has been banished from our diets!

As for that moderation myth . . .

Clearly, there's an abundance of scientific evidence showing that consuming high fructose corn syrup on a regular basis can not only make you fat, but subject you to a wide variety of ills. You might now begin to realize why looking for products labeled "no HFCS" is of more than casual importance to your family's long-term health and well-being.

Of course, the corn-refining industry, using such strategies as its "Sweet Surprise" campaign, has long tried to persuade us that HFCS is just fine when consumed "in moderation." Even if this were true, moderation can be a difficult thing to achieve with an ingredient that's been added to countless products, including many that we might never suspect of containing it. In fact, according to the USDA, an average American consumed an estimated 27 pounds of HFCS in 2014 alone![185]

No, *moderation* is more a word that would apply to our intake of old-fashioned cane sugar, which is now being once again used to sweeten various items that until recently contained HFCS (and which can be purchased in any store, unlike HFCS).

The fact that plain old cane sugar is a lot less hazardous to our health than HFCS doesn't mean we should be consuming it with abandon. However, back when sugar, or sucrose, was the prevalent sweetener in the American diet, nothing even close to the levels of certain health problems that have emerged since HFCS replaced it was seen in the general population—and science has now clearly shown that there's a connection. In fact, by making HFCS appear to be just another form of "sugar," we're effectively hiding from consumers the identity of one of the key culprits in the now unprecedented escalations of various life-threatening maladies.

So, instead of referring to HFCS-laden beverages as "sugary," perhaps we should really be calling them "sickeningly sweet."

New study uncovers the way HFCS triggers various disease

The question of why HFCS has been linked to so many health problems, ranging from heart disease and diabetes to ADHD and Alzheimer's, may now have been answered by a team of scientists from UCLA.

In what is described as the first study of how fructose consumption affects all the genes, pathways, and gene networks in the parts of the brain that control metabolism and brain function, researchers found that it can cause hundreds of genetic changes associated with various diseases.

After sequencing around twenty thousand genes in the brains of rats, the scientists identified more than 700 in the hypothalamus (which controls metabolism) and more than 200 in the hippocampus (which is associated with learning and memory) that had fructose-induced alterations—most of them comparable to genes in humans. Two of them were said to be the first genes in the brain to be affected by fructose in a way that causes a sort of chain reaction, resulting in damage to many others, according to Xia Yang, an assistant professor of integrative biology and physiology who helped lead the study.

The research team also discovered something else: those effects can be undone with a little help from docosahexaenoic acid, or DHA, a form of omega-3 found in flaxseed oil, walnuts, fruits, veggies, fish oil, and fish, especially wild salmon (not salmon that's been farmed). "DHA changes not just one or two genes; it seems to push the entire gene pattern back to normal, which is remarkable," Yang noted.

DHA, which supports learning and memory functions, is produced by brain cell membranes, but in amounts not nearly large enough to bring about those changes. Because of that deficiency, the amounts needed to reverse the effects of fructose have to come from dietary sources, noted Yang's coauthor, Fernando Gomez-Pinilla, professor of neurosurgery and a member of UCLA's Brain Injury Research Center, who compared food to a pharmaceutical compound in its effects on the brain.

Prior to this study, Gomez-Pinilla had determined that eating a diet high in fructose for an extended period of time impairs learning and memory by disrupting the ability of brain cells to communicate with each other. In the new study, which was posted at EBioMedicine, a website maintained by the journals *Cell* and *The Lancet*, researchers discovered more about the chemical process that fructose uses to turn genes on and off in the brain.

After the rats in the study were trained to escape from a maze, they were divided into three groups: one whose water was laced with fructose equivalent to about a daily liter of soda, the second given fructose-flavored water and a DHA-rich diet, and the third whose water contained neither fructose nor DHA.

After six weeks of being fed in this manner, the rats were returned to the maze, where the ones who received either plain water or fructose water with DHA added were clocked through about twice as fast as the ones in the group that received fructose water alone without the benefit of DHA. In addition, those on a high-fructose diet showed significantly higher levels of blood glucose, triglycerides, and insulin, all of which are linked to obesity and diabetes in humans.[186]

New research points to risks of a "fetal-HFCS syndrome"

Just when it seemed the flood of recent research about how HFCS affects our bodies and minds couldn't get any worse, two more studies released just prior to the completion of this book showed it can also jeopardize the future health of unborn babies.

In one study, presented at the annual meeting of the Society for Maternal-Fetal Medicine in February of 2016, pregnant mice were given either water or a fructose solution to drink. Their offspring, all of whom were fed regular chow, were then subjected to a series of tests once they became a year old. The study found that hypertension, insulin resistance, and obesity—all markers of metabolic syndrome—had developed in those exposed to prenatal fructose.

While done on mice, lead researcher Antonio Saad, MD, of the University of Texas Medical branch in Galveston called the study "an important indicator of the effect of the mothers' diet during pregnancy on the health of their children later in life," illustrating that "consuming high fructose during pregnancy puts the child at future risk for a variety of health conditions including obesity and the many complications it causes."[187]

In the second study, published in May 2016 in the journal *Scientific Reports*, researchers found that pregnant mice fed a high-fructose diet, in addition to having higher levels of triglycerides and uric acid, had smaller fetuses and larger placentas than those fed standard chow. This, according to senior author Dr. Kelle H. Molle of the Washington University School of Medicine in St. Louis, could lead to obesity and other health problem in adulthood due to the body's tendency to overcompensate.

Taking the study one step further, researchers then evaluated the fructose intake of eighteen pregnant women who had scheduled Cesarean deliveries and found similarities between the women and the mice who had a high fructose diet during pregnancy, including increased levels of uric acid.

The researchers noted that the outcome indicates "a novel mechanism by which increased fructose consumption can negatively affect maternal-fetal outcomes" and emphasizes "the potentially negative effects of high fructose diets in humans, in particular during pregnancy."

Know your badditives and how to avoid them:

HIGH FRUCTOSE CORN SYRUP

- Buy organic processed foods, which are HFCS-free, whenever possible.
- Steer clear of soft drinks and other sweetened beverages (except for specialty brands made with cane sugar and other truly natural ingredients, such as Reed's).
- Read labels on conventional foods. With HFCS found in products as diverse as beverages, mayo, and pickles, you can't automatically assume something doesn't contain it just because it's not sweet.
- Avoid products containing "fructose," which can be another term for a type of HFCS that's 90 percent fructose used in low-calorie jams, jellies, syrups, and other products. (We've even found it used in products that claim to have no HFCS.)

MEAT GLUE

Pink Slime's Far More Sickening Sibling

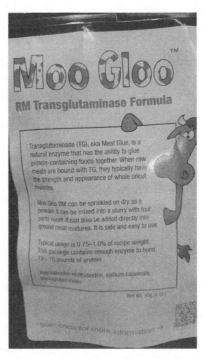

Moo-Gloo, one brand of transglutaminase, or "meat glue," is easily purchased online. The label states that it is "safe and easy to use." *Credit: Linda Bonvie*

"Meat is something you buy at your neighborhood local butcher shop. Glue is something you buy at Home Depot. Those two words just don't belong in the same sentence."[188]
— Grainne Trainor, owner, Blue Dining restaurant, McCandless, Pennsylvania

Back in 2012, an ABC news lead story about Pink Slime (called in the industry by the more appetizing name, "finely textured beef") struck a chord of disgust in the meat-eating public.

Petitions were formed to get the product out of the school lunch program, and celebrity chef Jamie Oliver conducted pink slime demos where he put beef scraps in a washing machine and then soaked them in ammonia and water.

Right before the slime hit the fan, however, ABC news affiliates spilled the beans about another underground meat practice. It was the use of an enzyme called transglutaminase, or, as it's more commonly referred to, meat glue.

Now, even though meat glue has the potential to be a lot more hazardous to your health than pink slime, for some reason, the public couldn't quite seem to wrap its head around it in the same way.

While some stories appeared in the press at the time, there were no petitions or consumers calling on the FDA or USDA to do something about it. In fact, some big-name chefs even came out in praise of meat glue.

For example, Wylie Dufresne, who was both chef and owner of the super-pricy Manhattan eatery wd~50 (which closed in 2014), was quoted in *Meat Paper* as saying he had "concocted all manner of playful and bizarre food products with meat glue, including shrimp spaghetti, which he made by mixing salt, cayenne, deveined shrimp, and meat glue in a blender."

"Meat glue," Dufresne declared, "makes us better chefs."[189]

However, even if you're dining at an elegant establishment like wd~50, you may want to think twice about eating "glued" food. That's one of the problems with this stuff—the appearance of food in which it has been used can definitely be deceiving.

How to fake a steak

This enzyme doesn't actually glue meat, chicken, or fish together like you might think a glue would work; instead, it interacts with protein to create a bond. Amino acids react with transglutaminase to become a sort of super glue that will hold up at the high temperatures in a grill or oven. It does its job so well you can't tell by just looking at a glued-together steak or piece of chicken or fish that it's not the real deal.

At one time, transglutaminase was manufactured entirely from the clotting agent extracted from pig or cow's blood. Now, it's typically made by cultivating bacteria to do the job. Most of the meat glue supplied to the food industry comes from none other than Ajinomoto—the company that brought MSG to America.

Like MSG, Ajinomoto claims that transglutaminase is "ubiquitous in nature . . . typically found in various plants and animals."[190] Where MSG is concerned, that premise really doesn't hold much water, as "bound" glutamic acid found in things such as meat, mushrooms, or tomatoes is quite different than the free glutamic acid added to food (see the chapter on MSG). Now, new research has found that this might also apply to transglutaminase sprinkled on meat or seafood (more on that in a moment).

What meat glue does is to allow restaurants and manufacturers to get away with one of the most devious forms of food fakery. Even the meat industry, when it defends transglutaminase, has to acknowledge that it can be used to fool diners. Meat glue is used much more often to "fake a steak" than to make gourmet shrimp noodles, as chef Dufresne did. By sprinkling the enzyme on various scrap pieces of meat, chicken, or seafood, and then binding it tightly in plastic wrap and refrigerating it for several hours, you can turn out a picture-perfect filet mignon, solid piece of chicken, or a top-dollar looking filet of fish.

Even experts can't tell the difference.

If you've ever attended a banquet or a convention, or maybe even dined in a restaurant, and were served an expensive-looking steak or sushi at a bargain price, you may have wondered how that came to be. The answer is either that the restaurant owner is losing money with each meal or, more likely, that there's a bag of meat glue in the kitchen.

A pathway for pathogens to get inside your dinner

Fakery aside, meat glue could be contributing to the growing epidemic of food poisoning that hits millions (the CDC puts the number at one in six Americans or around forty-eight million every year).[191]

That's because pathogens, like *Escherichia coli, Listeria*, and *Salmonella* (with many strains now antibiotic resistant) mostly appear on the surface of meat. When the outer surface is seared, even if the meat is eaten medium rare or rare, that bacteria has been killed.

When multiple pieces of meat are combined, however, those pathogens could be lurking in the center. Surfaces of the meat that once were on the outside are now in the middle. If you haven't cooked that meat thoroughly inside and out, you could be in for big trouble.

On an Australian TV exposé of meat glue several years ago, an expert in microbiology commented that "the amount of bacteria on a steak that's been put together with meat glue is hundreds of times higher" than your average piece of unglued meat.[192] The same is true for chicken and fish.

Now, if you ask the FDA, USDA, and certainly Ajinomoto, you're going to hear that meat glue is perfectly safe. Sure, there's that little problem of bacterial contamination, but these US consumer protection agencies appear to be quite confident that restaurants know that glued meat needs to be cooked thoroughly.[193]

The USDA calls it *TG enzyme*, and gives instruction for cooking stuck-together meat that sounds exactly the same as what it would tell you about cooking all types of raw meat. As far as the FDA is concerned, there's really no problem with Ajinomoto making its own determination that transglutaminase is generally recognized as safe, or GRAS.

Back in the late 1990s, the USDA received several petitions from both Ajinomoto and another company called AMPC about expanding the use of TG enzyme and attempting to get the consumer labeling (in the supermarket) to be as innocuous as possible.[194]

Both companies got just about everything they wanted. Meat glue can now be used in meat products across the board—both the kind the USDA calls "standardized" and "non-standardized." (This refers to what's called a "standard of identity"—a legal description of what it takes for certain foods to be able to use a name such as hot dogs, milk, cheese, bread, etc. For example, if you want to sell something called "Salisbury steak," it must contain at least 65 percent meat, among other requirements.)

In the case of meat glue, the agency had to *change* the standard of identity for numerous items like breakfast sausages, frankfurters, and bologna in order to allow for the use of the enzyme. Additionally, it was also approved to be used as a "binder" (something added to food to thicken or improve texture) for "certain meat and poultry products."[195]

As a result, it's quite possible that manufacturers are putting it to uses way beyond faking expensive cuts of meat.

Perhaps one of the most important reasons you need to go out of your way to avoid this badditive has to do with a more recent discovery—one that might help explain the explosion of gut and digestive troubles that are plaguing so many these days.

The role of meat glue in "tight junction dysfunction"

In 2015, researchers from Israel and Germany published a study on how "industrial food additives" could be the cause of the "rising incidence of autoimmune disease."[196]

Autoimmune diseases (when the body launches an attack on itself) have shown "strong evidence of a steady rise" in Western cultures over the last thirty years, the authors said. Cases of diseases such as type 1 diabetes, multiple sclerosis, Crohn's disease, lupus, and rheumatic and celiac diseases are climbing every year.

According to the researchers, these illnesses can be due to something called "tight junction dysfunction." Tight junctions refer to the "barrier and the fence" formed by connected cell membranes. When this finely tuned barrier is disrupted, it can set the stage for a wide variety of serious ailments.

The study, conducted by Professor Aaron Lerner and Dr. Torsten Matthias, called out transglutaminase as one of the commonly used food additives that can disrupt this internal barrier and enhance "intestinal junction leakage."

Additionally, like manufactured glutamic acid (MSG), the authors pointed out that TG enzyme is quite different from the transglutaminase found naturally in the human body. Its use in the food industry, they warn, is also expanding on a "great scale."

Celiac disease sufferers in particular, who are no doubt taking pains to avoid foods containing gluten, should also be aware of what these researchers believe is a link between their condition and meat glue, which may possibly explain the surge in celiac disease. "Several observations have led to the hypothesis that microbial transglutaminase is a new environmental enhancer of celiac disease," they noted in a 2015 report, explaining how the substance may affect the immune system and promote intestinal leakage, allowing "more immunogenic foreign molecules to induce celiac disease."

"If future research substantiates this hypothesis," they wrote, "the findings will affect food product labeling, food additive policies of the food industry, and consumer health education."[197]

In the meantime, however, consumers will remain on their own when it comes to protecting their health from this hazardous adhesive addition to their favorite dish—especially when dining out (and out of sight of what's being done in the kitchen).

Know your badditives and how to avoid them:

MEAT GLUE (TRANSGLUTAMINASE)

- When dining out, watch out for menu items that are priced so low they seem too good to be true—because they probably are. If you're attending a conference or convention, that rib-eye steak they're serving up may very well have been scraps of meat the day before (Remember: restaurants have no requirements for any kind of labels or warnings, so you pretty much have to trust the integrity of whatever establishment you patronize).
- Avoid buffet or supermarket "sushi." Good (and safe) sushi is an expensive and very skilled dish to prepare, but ersatz versions may well be put together with meat glue.
- If you're buying prepared meat, chicken, or seafood in the supermarket (either frozen or made into an entrée), check for either transglutaminase on the ingredient list or the words "formed" or "reformed" on the packaging. Don't expect to see any notice of this on the Nutrition Facts panel, which, in fact, is a very poor source of information about processed foods.

MSG AND ITS VARIOUS DISGUISES

The Hidden "Glutamic Bombs" in Our Food

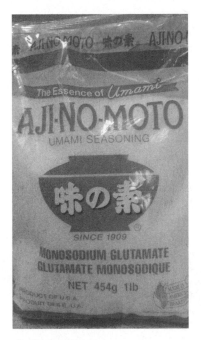

Credit: Linda Bonvie

"Why does the FDA allow the intentional addition of neurotoxic free glutamic acid (MSG) to processed food? Why isn't the US population aware of MSG's toxic potential? Why aren't healthcare professionals alert to the symptoms of MSG toxicity?"
—Adrienne Samuels, cofounder,
Truth in Labeling

The strange symptoms that investment banker and former hospital administrator Jack Samuels began suffering in 1989 had all the earmarks of Alzheimer's. As his wife Adrienne later recalled, they included "days of fatigue beyond imagination" and times when he "couldn't put a sentence together." However, "worst of all were the afternoons when he couldn't remember what he'd done in the morning."

While his doctor ruled out Alzheimer's, the cause remained a mystery. True, Jack had known for fifteen years that he was extremely sensitive to the flavor enhancer monosodium glutamate, but "this was something different." Besides, he and Adrienne were always scrupulously careful about avoiding anything that might contain the slightest amount of the additive.

Considering that Jack had put himself on a diet consisting of grapefruit, toast, and cottage cheese for breakfast; tuna fish on Wasa bread for lunch; and a slightly more varied, but insignificant, dinner, it didn't seem possible that any of those foods could possibly contain any MSG. However, after just two weeks of that seemingly bland regimen, he suddenly "lost his ability to speak in whole sentences."

It wasn't until the couple's oldest son suggested they read a book published the previous year by George Schwartz, MD called *In Bad Taste: The MSG Syndrome* that the cause of Jack's sudden affliction became obvious. Right there, on the cover, was the same tuna fish Jack had been eating every day for lunch.

The canned tuna, as it turned out, wasn't nearly as innocuous as it seemed. In addition to the actual fish and water, it contained an ingredient often added to tuna to make it taste better: hydrolyzed vegetable protein (HVP), which contains the same form of glutamic acid found in monosodium glutamate.* Glutamic acid just happens to be a neurotransmitter—a chemical that relays signals between nerve and brain cells (more on that in a moment).

HVP, the Samuels soon discovered, wasn't by any means the only such hidden form of MSG (the common acronym for monosodium glutamate, but one which can also be applied to other glutamate-based additives). Other ingredients in this category, which are routinely found in

---

* A scan of tuna fish cans in our local supermarket showed that HVP no longer seems to be used as an ingredient; however, "vegetable broth," which may be a source of MSG, can now be found in some canned tuna products.

a wide variety of processed food products, include calcium and sodium caseinate, autolyzed yeast, yeast extract, soy and whey protein concentrate and isolate, textured protein, and other "hydrolyzed" proteins, as well as things like malt extract, maltodextrin, bouillon, broth, and various types of seasonings or flavorings.

Once Jack Samuels eliminated the tuna fish, along with other similarly adulterated foods, from his diet, he lost his Alzheimer's-like symptoms, along with the frequent chest and joint pains and other symptoms he had suffered.[198]

For the rest of his life, however, he had to try as best as he could to avoid any foods that might be harboring such potentially devastating substances. His wife believes that the heart attack he suffered in November, 2011, which resulted in his death two months later at the age of seventy-six, might not have occurred "had he not spent half of the last quarter of his life fibrillating following ingestion of MSG hidden in food," as well as reacting to its presence in drugs he was given.[199]

In that regard, Jack Samuels was very much like the proverbial canary in the coal mine, and his ordeal resulted in the couple's founding of Truth in Labeling, an organization dedicated to identifying concealed sources of glutamic acid in processed foods that may be impacting the health of countless Americans, often without their realizing it. (Adrienne Samuels, who holds a PhD in research methodology, has chronicled all of this in a book entitled, *The Man Who Sued the FDA*.)

There is certainly no shortage of such sources. "In fact, pretty much any processed fast food is likely to contain added MSG, unless it specifically says otherwise," admits Phillip Broadwith, the business editor for *Chemistry World*, in a promotional pitch for glutamate. Only Broadwith's statement, which appears on the website of the Royal Society of Chemistry, is itself misleading. That's because many products that claim to have "no added MSG" actually do contain it in one or more of those disguised forms.[200]

What all of these foods have in common is that their taste is artificially enhanced. In a sense, they can be compared to athletes who use performance-enhancing drugs to artificially boost their scores. But whereas the practice of "doping" in sports is considered cheating, no such stigma is attached to the use of flavor enhancers to turn a cheap recipe or unenticing product into a "taste sensation" (as illustrated by a jingle for the standard supermarket brand of monosodium glutamate: "A little Accent, like a little love, surely helps.") While those who use anabolic steroids, human growth hormone, and other doping agents are usually aware of the risks involved, countless consumers who are being exposed every day to MSG in its various forms have no clue about the dangers these ingredients might pose to their health.

MSG-reaction denial: the industry ploy that puts numerous people at risk

"If it's not Stove Top, it's not Thanksgiving," went the slogan on a commercial in which an actor dressed as a pilgrim "faked an attack of scurvy" to get out of a Thanksgiving dinner that didn't include Stove Top.

Unfortunately, including this kind of stuffing in your holiday festivities might actually cause some dinner guests to suffer symptoms similar to his simulated scurvy attack. That's because two of its ingredients (at least when the commercial was aired in 2014) were monosodium glutamate and hydrolyzed soy protein, another source of free glutamic acid, both of which have been associated with a whole range of adverse reactions that include migraines, shortness of breath, nausea and vomiting, seizures, rage reactions, and atrial fibrillation, to name just a few.

The tendency to cause such immediate reactions in sensitive individuals is one of the things that distinguishes ingredients in the extended family of glutamate-based ingredients from most other badditives. While all such undesirable substances sooner or later tend to have disastrous effects on health and well-being, consuming these particular ones can act immediately to put many people out of commission and, in some cases, land them in the emergency room.

Of course, that can now be said of other types of food components as well, a common example being peanuts, to which many people are highly allergic these days (a reaction that was practically unheard of a few decades ago). The difference, however, is that whereas peanut allergies are now accorded a great deal of official recognition, with warnings displayed on product labels whenever peanut contents are present, MSG sensitivity has remained the Rodney Dangerfield of reactions in that it gets little or no respect from the FDA, health authorities, mainstream medicine, or the food industry.

Instead, any and all reactions to the many foods containing either monosodium glutamate or its various culinary cousins have long been relegated to the realm of "Chinese restaurant syndrome," a condition first coined in a 1968 letter from a doctor to the *New England Journal of Medicine,* in which the writer talked about his having developed certain apparent reactions to Chinese food (which often contains large amounts of MSG). The doctor's symptoms included numbness at the back of the neck that radiated to both arms and the back, general weakness, and palpitations, which lasted for about two hours. In fact, there seems to have been a systematic suppression of any and all information, whether research based or anecdotal, showing that the effects of these ingredients can often be far more serious than such transient and superficial symptoms.

The strategies used to downplay such adverse reactions by the Glutamate Association, an industry trade group, and others with a vested economic interest in keeping these insidious "flavor enhancers" in foods have taken a variety of forms, including:

- The use of industry-controlled research, researchers, and forums to "prove" how safe and harmless these ingredients are. A typical example of the deceptive methodology involved in this effort has been the use of placebo-controlled studies that have purportedly showed no difference in the way subjects reacted to ingesting monosodium glutamate or the placebos. Only those "placebos," as Samuels has noted, turned out to be laced with other sources of glutamic acid, such as autolyzed yeast or hydrolyzed protein, as well as the artificial sweetener aspartame, the effects of which can be quite similar to free glutamate[201] (a subject covered in the chapter on aspartame).
- Breaching the firewall that's supposed to exist between manufacturers and regulators. Dr. Schwartz cited one flagrant example he uncovered some years ago in the form of an FDA pamphlet that purported to give the facts about MSG safety. The publication, however, was actually the work of the Glutamate Association (and was taken out of circulation after Schwartz complained to FDA brass).[202] Samuels also recalls a time when the FDA responded to consumer concerns on the subject by referring questioners directly to the Glutamate Association or sending them its material.[203]

- Using advertising and other means to influence mainstream medical journals to publish industry-supported studies supporting the idea that MSG-based additives are really nothing to worry about, and having such flawed research peer reviewed by individuals with close ties to the industry.[204] In some cases, as neuroscientist Dr. John Olney, a leading authority on MSG safety issues, discovered, these kinds of studies appeared in journals that were "editorially controlled by the authors of the studies (or their cronies)."[205]

- Courting conventional medical practitioners (a technique commonly used by drug companies). Allergists, for instance, have proven very useful in maintaining MSG safety claims by citing results of standard (meaning IgE-mediated) allergy tests, rather than recognizing MSG sensitivity as a reaction to a neurotoxic substance.[206]

- Manipulating media to help reassure consumers of the safety of products containing MSG—and that anything they might read to the contrary was simply an unfounded "Internet rumor." The methods used to achieve this range from the strategic placement of advertising to sending out industry hype disguised as news, a time-honored technique of the public relations profession.

One example of the latter we encountered back in 2014 was a short article on the website of the supposedly objective *Washington Post* under the category "Speaking of Science," headlined, "No, MSG isn't bad for you." Accompanying it was a three-minute propaganda video produced by none other than the American Chemical Society, claiming that MSG is "perfectly safe for the vast majority of people" and that anything you may have heard about its "toxic, poisonous, energy-sucking, headache-inducing reputation" is nothing more than a "food myth"; in fact, "one of the biggest lingering food myths of all."[207] (It should be noted that while a nonprofit, the ACS has a "Board Committee on Corporation Associates (CA)" described on its website as "the formal link between the American Chemical Society and chemical and allied industries" with more than twenty-five companies actively participating and paying annual dues, and being given the chance to attend "briefings on Capitol Hill regarding related topics of interest to legislators and industry."[208] The individual members, who are chemists and not biologists or toxicologists, are likely employed by or affiliated with industry.)

The result of this ongoing campaign might be called "MSG-reaction denial"—a widespread refusal to acknowledge the immediate and often serious risks that products laced with free glutamic acid pose to many sensitive individuals. Only lately, some chinks have begun appearing in that industry-tailored suit of armor.

Take, for example, the ambiguous description of "Chinese restaurant syndrome" provided on the mainstream health website Medline-Plus. After making the standard claim that since the syndrome was first identified, "many studies . . . have failed to show a connection between MSG and the symptoms some people describe," which is why it continues to be used, it then adds the disclaimer: "However, it is possible that some people are particularly sensitive to food additives."

How sensitive? Well, sensitive enough, it appears, to result in "abnormal heart rhythm" as measured on an electrocardiogram, "rapid heart rate," and "decreased air entry into the lungs." While "most mild symptoms, such as headache or flushing, need no treatment," it warns that "life-threatening symptoms," which may include chest pain, heart palpitations, shortness of breath, and swelling of the throat, "require immediate medical attention."[209]

"As researchers, we don't yet know what percentage of the population is sensitive to MSG," observes Kathleen Holton, a professor at the American University's Center for Behavioral Neuroscience in Washington, DC. "But we do know enough to confirm that the amino acid glutamate, when in its free form (i.e., when it is not bound to a full protein like meat), causes negative reactions in certain people"— which she notes are not limited to those described as Chinese restaurant syndrome. In a double-blind, placebo-controlled study she did on the effects of MSG in individuals with irritable bowel syndrome and the chronic pain condition fibromyalgia, she observed that symptoms such as headache (including migraine), diarrhea, gastrointestinal pain and bloating, extreme fatigue, muscle pain, and cognitive dysfunction all improved when subjects were put on a diet low in free glutamate, and which returned with re-introduction of MSG.[210] One such reaction (though what researchers would call "anecdotal") was described by a woman identified as "Emily G." and posted at a message board maintained by the website Msgmyth.com. "I would suffer from extreme cramping abdominal pains about five hours after eating. I was in so much pain it was difficult to breathe, my chest would feel tight, and I would lie on the floor curled up as I tried to live through the pain in my abdomen." She told of seeing numerous doctors, who were unable to find anything that should be causing her such problems. However, after giving up foods containing MSG (and eventually all processed foods), her health improved dramatically. "I feel fantastic each and every day. I sleep well, I feel good, I love living like this," she said.[211]

One mainstream health organization warns of a reaction that could be quite serious. The American Heart Association specifically includes "eating MSG" on its list of "common 'triggers' that might lead to an episode" of atrial fibrillation, or AFib, a condition that makes you "five times more likely to have a stroke" and can also help lead to "eventual heart failure due to the weakening of the heart muscle."[212]

In other words, eating not just Chinese food but also any of the numerous products, ranging from snack foods to soups that contain free glutamic acid can indeed bring on some very severe, and even life-threatening, reactions in a certain percentage of people—only without their being given the benefit of any warning about its presence (unlike commonly acknowledged allergens such as peanuts). That's something that makes the campaign of official denial dangerously misleading.

The cozy alliance between regulators and the regulated

Google the meaning of "Inside the Beltway" and you'll come up with "an American idiom used to characterize matters that are, or seem to be, important primarily to officials of the US federal government, to its contractors and lobbyists, and to the corporate media who cover them—as opposed to the interests and priorities of the general US population."

Perhaps no better example of that definition exists than the "Alliance for a Stronger FDA," a partnership that goes far in explaining why the FDA can seem so maddeningly slow and reluctant to correct threats to the health and safety of the "general US population" such as that posed by the presence of flavor enhancers such as MSG.

The only thing about the organization that differs from various other inside-the-Beltway organizations, in fact, is that the media seem almost totally unaware of its existence. As Beltway insiders go, this particular one has succeeded in keeping a kind of low profile.

The Alliance does, however have an impressive list of dues-paying members—one made up of dozens of nonprofit groups, law firms, companies (nearly all pharmaceutical ones), and trade associations representing industries regulated by the very same FDA. Included among the latter are the American Bakers Association, the Independent Bakers Association, the American Frozen Food Institute, and the Snack Food Association—all representing sectors of the food industry that would be affected by any attempted reforms in what's considered GRAS and what isn't.

According to its website (www.strengthenfda.org), the Alliance has two goals: to assure that the FDA "has sufficient resources to protect patients and consumers," and 'to maintain public confidence and trust in the FDA." One has to wonder just how much confidence and trust the public can put in an agency that's allied with many of the same entities it's supposed to be regulating.

The Alliance's deputy executive director, Steve Grossman, doesn't view that as a problem. "Everybody who is overseen by the FDA benefits when the agency is seen as strong and competent and a gold standard for the world," he told one of the authors of this book who interviewed him back in 2011.

While on any given day members may have a complaint about something the FDA is doing, "they understand that their concerns won't be made better by the agency's having fewer resources," he added. One reason is that a regulatory body that's short on people "qualified to investigate the science and run the lab tests" is apt to "make the most conservative decisions because it doesn't want to do anything wrong."

Could that, do you suppose, be what accounts for the FDA's continued acceptance of badditives, such as MSG, despite the mounting body of scientific and empirical evidence that they are causing massive harm to human health? Might the agency be reluctant to ruffle the feathers of those in industry who support the idea of creating a stronger FDA by giving it added resources?

The great glutamate deception

One of the most deceptive assertions often heard in regard to food additives is that some aren't essentially any different from naturally occurring ingredients. That's especially true when it comes to the glutamic acid found in monosodium glutamate, hydrolyzed protein, sodium caseinate, and similar flavor enhancers. Typical is Broadwith's claim in *Chemistry World* that glutamate is "a natural component of proteins, and there is chemically no difference between 'natural' glutamate and that added in the form of industrially produced MSG."[213]

What's overlooked by such industry pitchmen is that there's a vast difference in the way the body handles the glutamate found naturally in foods like tomatoes, mushrooms, and aged cheese and the manufactured varieties that processed food manufacturers have been increasingly adding to their products for the past several decades.

After being introduced to the US food industry at a 1948 conference as an ingredient that had been used to fortify the flavor of rations given to Japanese soldiers, monosodium glutamate was soon being added to more and more of the products lining the shelves of US supermarkets. It was at first extracted from protein sources in a manner similar to the way it had been obtained from kombu in Japan, which was the form in which it was "grandfathered" into the list of GRAS (generally recognized as safe) ingredients under the 1958 Food Additives Amendment to the Food, Drug, and Cosmetics Act. It didn't stay that way for long. Instead, a new process of bacterial fermentation allowed it to be made much more cheaply and easily.[214]

In addition, a method was introduced of boiling vegetables deemed unsuited for sale in vats of acid, then neutralizing them in caustic soda to produce a brown sludge-like material containing MSG and two other harmful chemicals called "hydrolyzed vegetable protein, or HVP.[215] While no comprehensive tally has been kept of just how many products have since been laced with these ingredients, an idea can be gotten from a recall in the summer of 2010 due to a *Salmonella* outbreak, which included a total of 177 different items containing HVP that were made by one company alone.[216]

As such "new and improved" ingredients became standard in everything from soup to nuts, the reports of adverse health effects associated with them began to rapidly multiply. Predictably, such complaints have been categorically dismissed by industry representatives and supporters in the mainstream medical community, who have continued to maintain that glutamate is glutamate, whether found in a tomato or a potato chip. However, what they have consistently failed to take into account is the simple fact that the glutamates naturally found in foods are bound together with proteins, permitting them to be slowly absorbed into the system, whereas manufactured "free glutamate" is quickly assimilated, producing a corresponding spike in blood levels. (In this regard naturally occurring glutamates are quite similar to the fructose found in fruit as opposed to the "free fructose" added to products like high fructose corn syrup.)

Also, manufactured glutamic acid contains numerous chemical impurities, some of which are known to be carcinogenic. "The consequences of the interactions of these various chemicals with other chemicals and/or with the digestive processes are unknown," says Samuels. Their effects, scientists soon discovered, weren't merely limited to the growing list of symptoms that have ranged from numbness and headaches to the type of temporary cognitive impairments experienced by Jack Samuels.

The MSG–obesity connection

Could our cumulative consumption of MSG in its many forms be contributing to our current enormous obesity problem?

That seems likely, according to recent research into the neurobiological effects of these ingredients.

In one 2011 study, for instance, the dietary habits of more than ten thousand adults in China were scrupulously monitored for about five and a half years. The researchers found that those who ate the most MSG—averaging about five grams a day—were 30 percent more apt to be overweight than those who consumed the least—less than half a gram daily (actually, the figure is upped to 33 percent if we take into account those with excess body weight who were eliminated at the outset).

The results led to conjecture that MSG's effect on the hypothalamus may bring about overproduction of the hormone leptin, which is linked to appetite and metabolism, by causing leptin resistance. Or, using MSG to enhance the flavor of food could lead to overeating.[217]

Another study, this one done on mice by an international research team and published in the *Journal of Medicinal Food* in 2014, concluded that "MSG appears to be a critical factor in the initiation of obesity." The researchers, led by Makoto Fujimoto of the University of Toyama in Japan, noted that at twelve months of age, the mice fed MSG had "manifestations of obesity," whether they were fed a restricted or control diet.[218]

These and other findings serve to support earlier indications that all those MSG-based additives may well be part of the reason that more than a third of Americans are now considered overweight. As Dr. Blaylock put it nearly two decades ago, "One can only wonder if the large number of people having difficulty with obesity in the United States is related to early exposure to food additive excitotoxins, since this obesity is one of the most consistent features of the syndrome. One characteristic of obesity induced by excitotoxins is that it doesn't appear to depend on food intake. This could explain why some people cannot diet away their obesity."[219]

Are we short-circuiting our kids' brains?

In an age when attention deficit hyperactivity disorder, or ADHD, has become so prevalent that children are routinely prescribed drugs for it (with all the risks that entails), one has to wonder if this condition is a result of something different about the way kids are now being raised. And what about the growing epidemic of classroom violence? As we asked a number of years ago in a newspaper article we did on the subject, could what's eating kids be a result of what they're eating?

Based on what some experts on neurology and nutrition believe, there could well be a direct connection between food ingredients and behavioral problems that were virtually unheard of a few decades ago. While some of the badditives that may be at the root of much of these behavioral abnormalities are discussed in the chapters on artificial colors and preservatives, the likely role of excitotoxins is something that most attempts to analyze these developments fail to take into account.

Excitotoxins are neurotransmitters used as food ingredients that are capable of literally exciting certain brain cells to death when consumed in excessive amounts. These substances, according to neuroscientists, cause the neurons to be flooded with calcium, which activates them briefly under normal circumstances, but continues to do so when an excitotoxin is present, until they die.[220]

One type of excitotoxin is the artificial sweetener aspartame, containing the neurotransmitter aspartic acid, which is covered in a previous chapter. Another is the unbound glutamate that is found in all those MSG-based flavor enhancers.

A particularly frightening aspect of the scientific literature on MSG in its various disguises is the apparent damage these substances can do to the complex circuitry of the developing brain. In that sense, you might think of them as little "glutamic bombs"—tiny explosive charges whose effects may not be immediately evident, but are apt to become amplified in unpredictable ways.

The neurotoxic character of MSG was first discovered back in 1957 by two ophthalmologists in the course of using it on newborn mice that they were studying for a hereditary eye disease, only to find that the MSG had destroyed all the nerve cells in the inner layers of the animals' retinas. A decade later, Dr. John Olney, a neuroscientist at Washington

University in St. Louis, repeated their work, and made a further unsettling discovery—that a single dose of MSG was all it took to kill the cells in the hypothalamus, a critical part of the brain that regulates things like the onset of puberty, appetite, sleep cycles, the autonomic nervous system, and endocrine glands, and is part of the circuitry involved with feelings of rage and aggression.[221, 222] The hypothalamus, as Olney noted, is a part of the brain unprotected by the blood-brain barrier,[223] a biological mechanism that ordinarily protects most of the brain from toxins but isn't yet fully functional in children.

What made Olney's findings especially significant was the fact that substantial amounts of monosodium glutamate were then being added to baby food. However, in an attempt to alert the public about this invisible danger to the health of developing brains and galvanize the FDA into taking action, he ran into a brick wall of industry interests.

As prominent neurosurgeon and consumer advocate Dr. Russell Blaylock noted in his book, *Excitotoxins: The Taste That Kills*, the FDA relegated the matter to a "Food Protection Committee" whose members "seemed more interested in what the food industry spokesman had to say" than in the findings of a highly respected neuroscientist. When he looked into the committee's background, Olney soon discovered that "it was founded by, funded by, and totally controlled by the food industry."[224]

It was only when Olney took his case to a Senate committee that manufacturers finally began to feel enough heat to voluntarily remove the monosodium glutamate from jars of baby food in 1969; although, according to Blaylock, they continued to add hydrolyzed protein, a "hidden" source of three other excitotoxins, to baby food products for the next seven years.[225]

Although Dr. Olney's campaign may have succeeded in halting the most flagrant abuse in which the MSG purveyors engaged, it did nothing to curtail the widespread use of monosodium glutamate and other brain-damaging additives in numerous processed foods that were—and are to this day—being regularly fed to kids at very young ages. Additionally, many children are being exposed to these substances even before they're born when women consume them during pregnancy (such products "can readily cross the placental barrier and overstimulate the growing brain of the fetus," the late nutritionist Carol Simontacchi noted in her book, *The Crazy Makers*.[226])

What makes all this especially alarming, according to a survey taken years ago, is that while kids often consume the same amounts of MSG as adults (with the number of products containing it having grown considerably since then), a child's brain, according to Dr. Blaylock, is "four times more sensitive" to these toxins than an adult's. Or, as Olney once observed, "The amount of MSG in a single bowl of commercially available soup is probably enough to cause blood glutamate levels to rise higher in a human child than levels that predictably cause brain damage in immature animals."[227]

So, what impact might all that consumption of excitotoxins at a very young age be having on our kids today? In his book, Blaylock pointed out that children's brains go through a "critical period" of development for as long as six or seven years after birth, and that feeding them a steady diet of excitotoxins may be having "devastating effects" on that process. Such effects, he said, "might be subtle, such as a slight case of dyslexia, or more severe, such as frequent outbursts of uncontrollable anger." In fact, "injections of minute amounts of glutamate into the hypothalamus of animals has been shown to produce sudden rage." He also raises the possibility that such early exposure might result in seizures, autism, or schizophrenia and could even make someone prone to "episodic violence and criminal behavior in later years."

Those aren't the only potential unintended consequences of excitotoxins coming into contact with unprotected brain cells. The damage they cause may also set the stage for neurodegenerative disorders such as Alzheimer's, Parkinson's, and ALS. According to Blaylock, it isn't just children who are vulnerable to their effects on the brain, but many older people as well, especially those whose blood-brain barriers may have been compromised by strokes, brain injuries, drugs, or various health problems such as hypertension, thus increasing their risk of brain cell death or injury from eating foods containing these additives.[228]

In that respect alone, the symptoms suffered by the late Jack Samuels after eating that HVP-adulterated tuna fish may have been symptomatic of a far more insidious risk to the physical and mental health of the public than even those health officials willing to acknowledge the existence of some adverse reactions to MSG may ever have imagined.

The pervasiveness of these glutamatic bombs in our diet isn't the only threat excitotoxins pose to our brains and bodies. The use of the artificial sweetener aspartame in thousands of products creates a kind of double jeopardy that can easily compound the neurotoxic damage and amplify the range of adverse reactions they're capable of producing.

An object lesson in the importance of being an earnest ingredient label reader

An example of just how important it is to read product ingredient labels was a discovery we made back in 2014 as writers of the *Food Identity Theft* blogs for Citizens for Health—one that also demonstrates how food companies might be persuaded to recognize that getting rid of harmful additives is the right thing to do.

In checking out the ingredients of various products at our local supermarket (something we routinely did to keep readers informed), we found a snack food that we considered to be a potentially dangerous misrepresentation of a widely trusted product.

The name of the item in question, Herr's Old Bay Seasoned Potato Chips, together with the large depiction of a familiar container on the package, might have led a lot of consumers to believe that the chips inside were flavored with Old Bay Seasoning, a "unique blend of spices and herbs" that, according to its website, has been produced to its "original exacting standards" for over seventy years. So might a blurb on the right side, signed by company president Ed Herr, describing how, for more than thirty years, Herr's had "been seasoning fresh-cut potato chips with the classic blend of heat, sweet and savory known as Old Bay." Also included were a brief description of the seasoning's history, along with a recipe idea for "Delicious Herr's Old Bay Potato Chip Crab Cakes."

Making that assumption, as we learned from a scan of the actual ingredients listing on the back of the package, could well have been a serious mistake for many consumers. What actually gave these chips their enticing flavor was monosodium glutamate, an ingredient *not* present in Old Bay Seasoning (as its manufacturer, McCormick & Co., has made a point of assuring consumers), which consists of celery salt, (salt and celery seed) and spices, including mustard, red pepper and black pepper, bay (laurel) leaves, cloves, allspice (pimento), ginger, mace, cardamom, cinnamon, and paprika. Failing to realize that, as we noted at the time, might have landed someone who was particularly sensitive to the neurotoxic flavor enhancer in the ER.

What we really found startling was the explanation we received from a quality-assurance executive at Herr's: that the "total seasoning package" that went into Old Bay Potato Chips was supplied by McCormick, with his company being responsible only for the "base product" of sliced potatoes and some added salt.

"This is a formulation that came out quite a few years ago and hasn't been touched since," he told us. "The package design is one they encouraged us to have . . . they thought it was great for us to promote the product and Old Bay at the same time." However, he acknowledged that what the Old Bay Chips were seasoned with was "an entirely different product" than the Old Bay Seasoning sold in supermarkets.

While, like many people in the food industry, he claimed not to be concerned about monosodium glutamate based on its supposedly having come "under scrutiny by the FDA" and been given a GRAS rating, he did note that "our company and other companies are looking at ways to eliminate MSG, particularly in new products." He added, "What has been harder is [getting rid of it in] products that have been tremendously successful and are difficult to reformulate. This product is very successful, particularly in major markets where Old Bay Seasoning is popular."[229]

However, apparently it turned out to be not that hard to get rid of. The year after we ran this particular blog and a few follow-ups on this product (and a couple other Herr's "Old Bay Seasoned" snacks that also contained monosodium glutamate), we once again picked up a bag of those chips and were pleasantly surprised to find that the list of ingredients had been altered— and monosodium glutamate was no longer on it. In addition, mustard and celery had been newly listed as among the "spices" it contained in an apparent effort to make the seasoning more like the Old Bay blend.

If there's an object lesson here, it's that you should never take for granted that a product is free of MSG—or any other undesirable additive, for that matter—without checking the actual ingredient list. (Even organic products aren't totally exempt from this rule.) In other words, you shouldn't put anything in your mouth (and your stomach) without first knowing what's really in it!

(A post script to this little episode: As we were completing this book, we discovered a product in the supermarket we hadn't seen before: Herr's Old Bay Cheese Balls in a 19-ounce plastic bottle featuring a depiction of Old Bay Seasoning and containing—you guessed it—monosodium glutamate, along with two artificial colors. Sometimes, it seems like getting rid of badditives is almost like a game of whack-a-mole.)

Know your badditives and how to avoid them:

MSG

- Aside from avoiding processed foods that list monosodium glutamate on the label, watch out for *any* mention of hydrolyzed proteins, soy protein, soy protein concentrate and soy protein isolate, autolyzed yeast, sodium caseinate, textured protein, and yeast extract.
- For a more complete list of processed food ingredients that contain MSG, check out the Truth in Labeling page here: http://truthinlabeling.com/hiddensources.html.
- Don't rely on food labels that say "No MSG." Such products often contain one (or more) of the many aliases listed above.

PARTIALLY HYDROGENATED OILS

The Final Act of a Trans Fat Tragedy

Credit: Ryan Morrill Photography

"The use of partially hydrogenated vegetable oils in the American food supply has contributed to a national epidemic of coronary heart disease, causing tens of thousands of excess deaths each year and billions of dollars of additional health care expenditures."
—Dr. Fred Kummerow, professor emeritus,
University of Illinois

Consider for a moment the cost in human lives of three of the best-known tragedies of modern times. When the luxury liner *Titanic* sank in the North Atlantic in 1912 after hitting an iceberg, the official tally of passengers and crew members who died was 1,517. Japan's December 1941 attack on the American fleet in Pearl Harbor killed some 2,402 people all told, including several dozen civilians. When the United States was attacked by terrorists on September 11, 2001, the death toll, which included people inside the World Trade Center, the Pentagon, and the four hijacked airliners, was put at 2,996. When combined, the total number of people who perished in those three catastrophic events was 6,915.

Now, add another 85, and you've got the approximate number of Americans said to be dying *every year* in an ongoing disaster of a far different sort—the great trans fat tragedy.

These are the hidden victims of the industrial trans fats found in partially hydrogenated oils, or PHOs, which are oils that have been solidified via an infusion of hydrogen gas. Such oils have long been routinely added to a variety of processed foods to improve their texture and "flavor stability" and prolong their shelf life—even as they cut short the lives of those consuming them.

If you think the comparison offered above is somewhat of an exaggeration, it's actually based on figures provided by the US Food and Drug Administration—an agency hardly given to hysteria or hyperbole when talking about additives it has long allowed to be used in our food supply. According to an FDA estimate, that one ingredient alone is responsible for approximately 20,000 heart attacks and 7,000 related deaths per year.[230]

Of course, what makes the trans fat tragedy different is that it strikes people down one by one, with neither media coverage nor even any formal recognition of the real, underlying cause of their demise. While a victim's death certificate might attribute their passing to "coronary artery disease," for example, it won't mention those boxes and boxes of Girl Scout Cookies they consumed, which listed "partially hydrogenated oil" among their ingredients.

That's the bad news.

The good news is that after decades of so many commonplace products being laced with these artery-clogging materials, the FDA has finally ordered the PHOs that contain trans fats to be removed from the "generally recognized as safe (GRAS)" list and from most everyday food products by no later than June 18, 2018. "This action responds, in part, to citizen petitions we received," notes the agency's decree, adding that the determination was based "on available scientific evidence and the findings of expert scientific panels establishing the health risks associated with the consumption" of trans fat.[231] (The trans fat issue here, incidentally, is the kind added in the form of PHOs, and should not be confused with relatively small amounts of naturally occurring trans fat found in dairy products and meat from grass-fed cows, such as conjugated linoleic acid [CLA]. Research has found this form to have "potent anti-atherosclerotic effects,"[232] meaning that it's actually apt to be beneficial in reducing plaque buildup in the arteries.)

Up until that deadline, however, and likely even beyond it, you will still find partially hydrogenated oil listed as an ingredient in a variety of processed products, from baked goods to frozen foods. Even afterward, there may be numerous exceptions to the new rule, which the Grocery Manufacturers Association has indicated it hopes to wheedle out of the FDA.[233]

In fact, the pending prohibition on the further use of PHOs in grocery items has actually been a long time coming—and it hasn't come easy, by any means.

The long good-bye

While trans fats were first recognized as a cause of heart disease in the 1990s, it wasn't until 2006 that the FDA required that they be listed on Nutrition Facts panels. That, however, came with a major loophole for manufacturers, which allowed anything measuring less than 0.5 grams to be "rounded out" to 0, a provision that quite literally categorized substantial amounts of this potentially deadly goop as being "nothing to worry about" on the government's official guide to consumers.

Even after the FDA finally got around to proposing a ban in November of 2013, under pressure from consumer advocates (and one in particular, as we shall see), it took another year and a half for the agency to announce a schedule for implementing it.

Why the delay? Given the agency's own acknowledgment of the role PHOs have played in the mortality rate from heart disease (to say nothing of the cost of caring for heart attack and stroke survivors), shouldn't this proposal have been at the top of the order of business, with an "urgent" light flashing?

One might think so. But while the FDA may have been set up with a mission of protecting consumers, the industries it's supposed to regulate also wield a certain amount of influence over its decisions. This particular mandate did not come about without encountering a significant amount of resistance from Big Food. (In fact, much of its seventy-nine-page "final determination" on the matter was dedicated to addressing some of the objections raised by industry members or supporters, which were among the six thousand or so responses to the original proposals.)[234]

The Grocery Manufacturers Association (GMA), for example, urged the agency to support a "prudent" and "less onerous proposal," lest the food supply be significantly disrupted and consumers "unjustifiably denied access to products such as baked goods, pastries, confectioneries, some flavors, seasonings, and many other products." (The GMA, however, seems to have since found ways to cope with such disruption and denial, having responded to the actual ban by declaring that it "minimizes unnecessary disruptions to commerce.") [235]

Similarly, Mark B. Andon, vice president of research, quality, and innovation at ConAgra Foods, contended that dropping the GRAS status of PHOs "would place potentially thousands of food products at risk of being deemed adulterated due to the presence of an ingredient that has been safely and commonly used in foods for over fifty years."

Given the growing body of scientific evidence to the contrary, one can only assume that such a purported half century of safe use is based on nothing more than the idea that consumers haven't instantly keeled over and died upon eating PHO-laced products (as seems to be the case with other such "safety" claims as well).

Then there was the opinion expressed by food giant General Mills that "current low intakes of trans fat are safe" and that a level of trans fat below 0.2 grams per serving either be established as the new "zero" (a suggestion echoed by the American Bakers Association) or become a "threshold limit." Never mind that back in 2002, the National Academy of Science's Institute of Medicine determined that there is *no amount* of trans fatty acid that is actually "safe" to consume, declining to declare a safe upper limit, which it had the option of doing.[236] (It was that conclusion, in fact, that prompted the FDA to require that trans fat levels—the 0.5 loophole aside—be included on Nutrition Facts labels.)

Such responses, of course, were quite predictable. Back in 2006 when eateries in New York City were ordered to refrain from using trans fats in preparing food, the National Restaurant Association responded by calling the action, initiated by health-conscious Mayor Michael Bloomberg, "a misguided attempt at social engineering by a group of physicians who don't understand the restaurant industry."[237]

If anything, the fact that it took nearly a decade for the FDA to enact a similar ban in regard to processed foods tells you something about the reluctance of federal regulators to take on powerful corporate vested interests, even after it's become quite apparent that the practice in question is having a disastrous impact on the health and longevity of the population.

Not that the food industry, seeing the proverbial handwriting on the wall, didn't take some steps on its own during that period to curtail the use of PHOs in its products. Or at least it did, according to GMA spokesman Roger Lowe, who claimed it had already cut the use of added trans fats by 86 percent at the time of the FDA edict.[238] If that's true, it only goes to show just how much of these circulatory system–cloggers it must have previously been using, as indicated by a New York Department of Health analysis concluded less than a year earlier (nine months after the FDA initially proposed its ban). That study found PHOs in one out of every ten of the processed foods on grocery store shelves—84 percent of which were labeled as having "0 trans fats" thanks to that aforementioned FDA loophole![239]

Could consuming trans fats translate into poor test results?

As if it wasn't bad enough that consuming foods with PHOs substantially increases your risk of dying from a heart attack, they have also been found capable of messing up your memory.

In late 2014, a research team from the University of California in San Diego tested the memories of more than a thousand young and middle-aged men after having them fill out questionnaires about their dietary habits. The amount of trans fat that each subject ordinarily consumed could be estimated from the information they provided.

The subjects were then given a "recurrent word" test in which they were asked to remember whether certain words had already been shown to them on a series of 104 flash cards. When the results were compiled, it was found that the ones who ate the most PHOs could recall 11 or 12 fewer words than their peers, even when other factors were taken into account.

Study author Dr. Beatrice Golomb, a professor of medicine at the college, described that as "a pretty big detriment to function," given that the average number of words accurately recalled was 86. In fact, the researchers were able to estimate that every additional gram a day of trans fat consumed resulted in 0.76 fewer words committed to memory.

Now admittedly, this was only circumstantial evidence—an "association" between trans fat and memory loss, rather than direct proof. But it was enough to cause Golomb to characterize them as "metabolic poisons" whose energy-sapping oxidative effects can effectively put brain cells that retain memories out of commission.

"Trans fats were most strongly linked to worse memory in young and middle-aged men during their working and career-building years," she added.

Or, as Walter Willett from the Harvard School of Public Health in Boston put it, "these artificial fats penetrate every cell in the body and can disrupt basic cell functions."

(Interestingly enough, what inspired the UCSD team to conduct this study was a finding that eating chocolate actually seems to enhance our ability to remember. Since chocolate is an antioxidant that "supports cell energy" in the hippocampus, the part of the brain most associated with memory, it caused the researchers to wonder whether trans fats, which are known to cause oxidation in cells and deplete their energy, might have the opposite effect.)[240]

The saturated fat subterfuge

Of all the strategies attempted by the food industry in its efforts to deflect a ban on PHOs in food, the saturated fat subterfuge was perhaps the most deceptive. This particular ploy was exemplified in comments made by Matt Jansen, senior vice-president of Archer Daniels Midland Co. and president of its global oilseeds and cocoa business, who claimed that a PHO ban "would inevitably lead to increased use of fats and oils higher in saturated fatty acids, making it more difficult for consumers to comply with the Dietary Guidelines recommendations on saturated fat intake."

In other words, removing trans fats would cause people to consume other unhealthy forms of fat. That's not only speculative; it's also based on a badly outdated notion regarding the health effects of saturated fats, such as those found in butter. In fact, around the same time that comment was submitted, a comprehensive review of seventy-two studies from eighteen countries undertaken by researchers from Britain's University of Cambridge determined that saturated fats do not pose an increased cardiac risk after all.

This wasn't the only research to reach such a conclusion. In August of 2015, just two months after the FDA delivered its long-overdue ultimatum to the food industry on PHOs, another study out of McMaster University in Ontario, Canada, compared the risks of consuming trans fats with those of eating saturated fats. It, too, supported previous findings that trans fat consumption can significantly increase the likelihood of heart attacks, and in fact up the risk of suffering a fatal one by a full 28 percent. But it found no clear indication of a link between saturated fats and cardiovascular disease (CVD), coronary heart disease (CHD), ischemic stroke, type 2 diabetes, or, for that matter, death from any cause.

Actually, the long-held idea that foods rich in natural fats were major contributors to heart disease mortality statistics was what helped bring about the trans fat intrusion on our diet in the first place. The acceptance of those trans fats, in turn, further misled the people involved in formulating our nutritional guidelines into mistaking the "good guys" for "bad guys"—and vice versa.

A brief historical perspective offers some illumination into how a topsy-turvy misapprehension of this magnitude can evolve into conventional wisdom, and remain that way for such a long period of time.

In fact, that's how this whole fiasco started—not with food, but with illu-mination. That is to say, not with bakers, but with candle makers.

Back around the end of the nineteenth century, the folks who man-ufactured soap and candles began looking for substances to substitute for lard and tallow, whose prices were controlled by the meat-packing industry. Enter E. C. Kayser, a German chemist who sold Procter & Gamble on a way of turning liquid cottonseed oil into a solid similar in consistency to lard via the process of hydrogenation.

This happened around the same time that electric lighting was greatly reducing the need for candles. As companies so often do under such cir-cumstances, P&G began looking for new uses of its hardened cottonseed oil product—and eventually found one. Given its lard-like appearance, the company decided it would make a dandy grease for cooking. The resulting product, first introduced in 1911 and named Crisco, a play on crystallized cottonseed oil, only needed a catchy claim and slogan to convince housewives to use it instead of more traditional commod-ities. That's where P&G's marketing geniuses came in, hyping it as an all-vegetable shortening that was "a healthier alternative to cooking with animal fats . . . and more economical than butter."[241]

Of course, there were no scientific studies at the time that validated any such health claims—but in those days, a lot of such unproven assertions were made for products. (One of the reasons the FDA was established, in fact, was to create legitimate standards for this chaotic marketplace.) In this case, however, the idea took hold and remained unchallenged through most of the twentieth century.

A number of factors contributed to that misconception's perpetuation, the first being the publication of a 231-page cookbook in 1913 called *The Story of Crisco,* which included 615 recipes all calling for the use of the shortening, and which was given out by the company. As described by food writer Linda Joyce Forristal, the book presented Crisco as "healthier, more digestible, cleaner, more economical, more enlightened, and more modern than lard," with the women who used it "portrayed as good wives and mothers" whose houses were free of strong cooking odors and whose children grew up with good characters. That wasn't all. As Forristal notes, P&G also convinced Jewish housewives that the shortening was better than butter in that it could also be used in preparing meat dishes (the mix-ing of meat and dairy products being forbidden under religious dietary law). This resulted in their switching not only to Crisco but also to margarine "more quickly than other groups, with unforeseen consequences."[242]

The spreading of margarine mania, in fact, was what one might call the dropping of the other trans fat shoe. Initially introduced in 1869 in France as the winning entry in a competition held by Emperor Napoleon III to find a cheaper substitute for butter, and subsequently refined by the Dutch, this imported imitation was subject to all kinds of restrictions at the behest of the dairy lobby. At one time, it could not be legally sold in more than half the states, while others forbade coloring it yellow so it resembled butter, mandating that margarine manufacturers dye their product pink instead (prompting some to sell it along with a separate package of food coloring that could be added at home).

Eventually, however, butter shortages during both world wars brought about an easing of such restrictions, and as American consumers began using margarine and realized that it was both cheaper and easier to spread than butter, its appeal increased, and legislators were urged to "repeal anti-margarine laws." Finally, in 1950, Congress voted to do away with a margarine tax that was the last major obstacle to its widespread substitution for butter.[243]

In the years that followed, as neurobiologist and obesity researcher Stephan Guyenet has noted, margarine largely came to replace butter in our national diet, reaching a point in 1975 where Americans were eating only a quarter the amount of butter and ten times the amount of margarine they consumed in 1900.[244]

But that's not surprising, given that consumers were constantly being told that margarine was a heart-healthy product, and butter a culinary culprit whose saturated fat content was largely responsible for the rise in heart disease (along with cholesterol-rich eggs). And in the forefront of the crusade to curtail consumption of saturated fats was Dr. Ancel Benjamin Keys, a University of Minnesota scientist who, beginning in 1958, led a "Seven Countries Study" of nearly thirteen thousand men (although he ended up using results from just a few dozen) in the US, Europe, and Japan—a study whose results he claimed linked such fats to heart disease.

That conclusion would remain a mantra of mainstream medicine for decades after its publication, despite a number of significant shortcomings that were subsequently discovered in Dr. Keys' methodology (for example, focusing on residents of Crete during Lent, for which they had given up eating meat and cheese, while failing to include countries such as France and Switzerland where fat consumption was high and heart disease low). The anti-butter bias (which also helped spread margarine's reputation as a healthy alternative) really took root when the American Heart Association put saturated fats on its undesirable list after naming Dr. Keys to its nutrition committee in 1961.[245]

That was around the same time that processed food manufacturers, perhaps buoyed by the popularity of both Crisco and margarine, began to realize what the hydrogenation process could do for their bottom line (especially in regard to keeping products on shelves longer). PHOs suddenly began to appear on the ingredient lists of an increasing number of processed foods (not that many consumers were aware of their presence, let alone the damage they could inflict).

Guyenet believes that both the decrease in butter use and the rise in trans fat consumption have "contributed to the massive incidence of CHD seen in the US and other industrial nations today." He also points out that France, which has the highest per capita dairy fat consumption of any industrial nation, as well as a comparatively low intake of hydrogenated fat, "has the second-lowest rate of CHD, behind Japan."[246]

Maybe that's because, contrary to everything we were once led to believe, butter actually contains various antioxidants, such as vitamins A and E and selenium, which protect the health of your heart, while helping to strengthen the immune system and ward off diseases like cancer and osteoporosis. Until recently, however, misguided and unwarranted warnings from health officials were having the effect of depriving people of these very benefits, steering them toward counterproductive substitutes that not only included margarine but also less-than-healthy cooking oils.

Margarine claims of past years reflect how our 'fatitudes' have changed

"Should an 8-year-old worry about cholesterol?"

That was the question posed in a full-page 1971 ad for Fleischmann's Margarine in *Woman's Day* (one we would have showed you, had not ConAgra, which now owns the brand, refused us permission to reproduce).

The ad, which features a Normal Rockwell–type picture of a child in bed with his baseball hat and glove, warns how "cholesterol can start building up in a kid. Up and up, until he grows up with a real health risk." That was why it was so important to introduce your family to foods like Fleischmann's Margarine, with 100 percent corn oil, that were "low in saturated fat" and "high in polyunsaturates . . . to help reduce serum cholesterol."

Actually, that claim was a bit much for even the Federal Trade Commission, which asked the company to "tone down" its advertising, according to food historian Harvey Levenstein The FTC, he noted, ordered Fleischmann's to desist from claiming that its product could prevent heart disease, but did allow it to say that "it can be used as part of a diet to reduce serum cholesterol, which can contribute to the mitigation of heart and artery disease," because it was a good idea to acquaint consumers with some of the steps they could take to avoid heart disease.[247]

At the time, no one was worrying about the PHO in margarine and the resulting trans fat content. Even thirteen years later, a *New York Times* "guide for consumers" comparing the merits of various margarine brands, claimed that "the ratio of polyunsaturated to saturated fats is the key health consideration in margarine." It also referred to "the process of hydrogenation" as one that turned "some of the unsaturated fat to saturated," without making any mention of the trans fats it created. It further contended that "[m]any health professionals believe that to prevent a variety of illnesses, including heart disease, the lowering of overall fat consumption is more important than a change in the type of fat in the diet."[248]

Of course, we know better these days—sort of.

"In response to concerns about trans fat, we have developed Fleischmann's soft spreads to be trans fat-free," the company declares at a website it maintains. However, at that same site you'll also find "original spread" (both salted and unsalted,) whose Nutrition Facts panel notes that a serving contains 1.5 grams of trans fat.[249]

Vindication at 100

The year before Dr. Keys began his much-hyped study, another aca-
demic, Fred Kummerow, a professor of comparative biosciences of the
University of Illinois, was publishing a discovery of a quite different
nature. Having convinced a local hospital to let him examine the arteries of patients who had died of heart attacks, Kummerow was startled
to find that they were clogged with fat—not the saturated kind, but the
variety found in margarine and trans fats.

Kummerow then performed follow-up studies that showed such fats
had similar effects on laboratory animals. Only this time, he had some
good news for people who stopped eating them. "In 1958," he later wrote,
"I showed that if I fed a rat trans fat and then took it out of the diet, in
a month, the trans fat is . . . metabolized out. There's no more trans fat
in the body." He then commenced a campaign to have these substances
removed from the food supply, which he was convinced would result in
a decrease in the rate of "sudden deaths." He was, in fact, somewhat successful in getting the amounts reduced in margarines and shortenings
from 43 to 27 percent while serving on an AHA subcommittee in 1968,
a reduction he believes may have saved many lives. But it took another
half century for the FDA to finally take the kind of action he had been
pushing for.

Fortunately—and perhaps to some degree because he practiced
what he preached—Kummerow has lived long enough to see the practice of adding PHOs to food products finally about to come to an end.
In fact, he had already turned a hundred years old when the FDA got
around to proposing the ban that he, more than anyone else, appears
to have been responsible for bringing about (Kummerow likes to
recount how he threw out a ready-made cake someone unthinkingly
brought to his hundredth birthday party after he looked at the label
and saw it contained added trans fat, as so many store-bought confections do.[250]).

In 2009, Kummerow filed a three-thousand-word citizen petition
with the FDA that began, "I request to ban partially hydrogenated fat
from the American diet." Then, after waiting four years for a response, he
followed that up by filing suit against both the FDA and its parent bureau-
cracy, the Department of Health and Human Services, demanding that

PHOs be removed from the food supply unless new evidence of their safety should be found by a complete administrative review. In addition to charging that their continued use in the American diet had caused "as many as 100,000 excess deaths per year," his twenty-seven-page legal brief also asserted that the artificial trans fats they created were also resulting in diseases like type 2 diabetes, cancer, and Alzheimer's.[251] The agency's provisional revocation of GRAS status for these oils was announced a mere three months later.

In the meantime, Kummerow, in articles for peer-reviewed journals, has been busy sounding the alarm about the oxidation that results when supposedly "healthy" polyunsaturated oils, like soybean and corn oil, are used in frying, claiming that "cholesterol has nothing to do with heart disease, except if it's oxidized." (He has also authored two books, *Cholesterol Won't Kill You, But Trans Fat Could* and *Cholesterol is Not the Culprit: A Guide to Preventing Heart Disease*.)

There is one particular oil he feels comfortable recommending for cooking. "Coconut oil is okay to use because it has very little unsaturated fatty acid," he told us in an email.

Kummerow is not the only contemporary expert to suggest that coconut oil (not just any coconut oil, but the extra virgin and unrefined kind) be substituted for other cooking oils that for years have been misleadingly proclaimed as "healthy."

It wasn't so long ago, however, that coconut oil, like butter, was being condemned as a virtual cardiac menace, even though there was ample evidence to indicate otherwise.

The case of the compromised coconut oil

A couple decades ago, Michael Jacobson, head of the Center for Science in the Public Interest, was quoted as saying that "theater popcorn ought to be the Snow White of snack foods, but it's been turned into Godzilla by being popped in highly saturated coconut oil."

In retrospect, however, we now know that the chief of what's often been referred to as the "food police" had misidentified the monster that was actually responsible for any number of heart disease deaths and wrongly implicated an innocent party. We're not talking about the theater popcorn itself, but that "highly saturated coconut oil."

Jacobson's accusation, however, wasn't entirely wrong either. That's where the whole issue gets a bit muddled. Because while the CSPI head was simply reiterating a prevalent, if misguided, belief among experts at the time—that saturated fats were the things that were driving up heart disease rates (see box)—the particular coconut oil in question may indeed have been part of the problem. Here's why: according to Dr. Thomas Brenna, a professor of nutritional sciences at Cornell University, "most of the studies involving coconut oil were done with partially hydrogenated coconut oil, which researchers used because they needed to raise the cholesterol levels of their rabbits in order to collect certain data."

On the other hand, "virgin coconut oil, which has not been chemically treated, is a different thing in terms of a health risk perspective," Brenna noted. So, if that theater popcorn was indeed "Godzilla," it wasn't the coconut oil it was popped in per se that stigmatized it in this manner, but rather the fact that the coconut oil used had actually been turned into a PHO.[252]

Once having been cleared of that erroneous bad rap, coconut oil, like butter, is now being widely hailed by an increasing number of nutrition experts as an actual hero of heart health that's rich in beneficial medium-chain triglycerides. Something that's been known for quite a while, in fact, is that Polynesian populations of atolls in the South Pacific who regularly consume large amounts of virgin coconut oil have been found to be remarkably free of heart disease.

According to the abstract of a study published in 1981 in *The American Journal of Clinical Nutrition*, "the habitual diets of the toll dwellers from both Pukapuka and Tokelau are high in saturated fat but low in dietary cholesterol and sucrose," with coconut being the chief source of energy for both groups. While the Tokelauans, who consumed almost twice as much saturated fat from coconut as the Pukapukans, had a 35 to 40 percent higher rate of serum cholesterol, "vascular disease is uncommon in both populations and there is no evidence of the high saturated fat intake having a harmful effect in these populations"[253] (a finding that would seem to support Dr. Kummerow's conclusion that cholesterol itself "has nothing to do with heart disease").

Virgin coconut oil is also about 50 percent lauric acid, which kills pathogens and helps prevent bacterial, viral, and fungal infections. Its medium-chain triglycerides (MCTs) have also been shown to help promote weight loss both by increasing the burning of calories and decreasing hunger, to name a few of the other health benefits associated with it.[254] Additionally, in a 2004 study published in the journal *Neurobiology of Aging*, those MCTs were found to improve cognitive function in adults with memory problems—after only a single dose![255] To "sweeten the pot," it has an extremely pleasant flavor and aroma that enhances the appeal of any food you might fry or bake with it.

It's unfortunate that some of the supposed nutrition authorities who helped perpetuate such false negatives and based dietary guidelines on them have been understandably reluctant to admit that they have been repeatedly shown to be erroneous. In fact, it wasn't until 2015 that eggs were finally exonerated, along with other cholesterol-rich foods, by the government's Dietary Guidelines Advisory Committee, which stated that "having found no appreciable relationship between consumption of dietary cholesterol and serum cholesterol during its review of the relevant research," it had "determined that cholesterol is not a nutrient of concern for overconsumption."[256] Making that concession, you can be sure, wasn't easy, having caused a lot of supposed experts to end up with egg on their collective faces.

The bottom line is that while trans fats in the form of added PHOs have at last been officially recognized as "bad guys" that may have caused countless people to die prematurely, it may take a bit longer still for all those in the mainstream health establishment to finally concede that the saturated fats in commodities like butter and coconut oil are actually "good guys."

The good news is that just as many consumers realized they should eliminate PHOs from their diet years before the FDA got around to removing them from the food supply, it isn't necessary to wait for the entire health establishment to recognize how wrong it has been about saturated fat.

The scientific evidence is already well established—and being reinforced every year. As the old saying goes, "knowledge is power"—and in this case, it is the power to improve and preserve your health and prospects for longevity.

The unanticipated irony of an old sitcom satire on the non-fat fad

Back in 1993, when a classic episode of the TV sitcom *Seinfeld* entitled, "The Non-Fat Yogurt" was originally televised (now seen in reruns), no one probably realized how close it would come to demonstrating that old adage, "many a truth is said in jest."

The main story line involves the sudden popularity of a new non-fat frozen yogurt store, which Jerry, Elaine, and Kramer begin patronizing regularly—that is, until they all realize that they've inexplicably begun gaining weight. How could this be, when the only new thing they've been eating is that fat-free yogurt? Finally, Jerry takes it upon himself to have the yogurt in question tested, only to find that it does indeed contain fat after all. From this point, the show goes on to include a spoof on New York City politics, as then-mayoral candidate Rudolph Giuliani discovers his cholesterol count has gone through the roof, and the "non-fat yogurt scandal" suddenly erupts into a major campaign issue.

What the episode was really satirizing, however, was the obsession at that time with non-fat dairy products—which, in a somewhat ironic development, recent research has found may actually make people more prone to obesity and the diabetes that frequently accompanies it compared to products from which no fat has been removed.

It just so happened that in the same year the *Seinfeld* episode first aired, researchers began tracking some eighteen thousand middle-age volunteers in the Women's Health Study, all of whom were normal in weight and not suffering from cardiovascular disease, cancer, or diabetes at the outset. What they have now determined is that eating high-fat dairy products made participants eight percent less apt to become obese.

"We saw less weight gain for higher total dairy and high-fat dairy intake and also a lower risk of becoming overweight and obese in those who consumed more high-fat dairy," noted Susanne Rautiaine, the author of the study who is a research fellow at both Brigham and Women's Hospital and Harvard Medical School.[257]

Even more dramatic were the results of another study, done over the course of fifteen years and published in the journal *Circulation*, in which a Tufts University research team found that regular consumers of full-fat dairy products had a 46 percent lower risk of becoming diabetic than those who chose skim milk, low-fat cheese, and—yes—low-fat yogurt. That research was based on an analysis of their blood for biomarkers of such fat.

The latter study's results, according to its author, Dr. Dariush Mozaffarian, Dean of Tufts Friedman School of Nutrition Science and Policy, "suggest that national guidelines that focus only on low-fat dairy should be re-examined."[258]

The fact that Americans are still urged to follow such guidelines, despite mounting scientific evidence that saturated fat content in food is not the health hazard it was hysterically proclaimed to be a quarter century or more ago, is of course a reflection of the reluctance to let go of concepts on which both so-called experts and respected institutions have staked their reputations.

These latest findings, if nothing else, are a further example of how, more and more, the conventional wisdom that has driven so many of our ideas about health and nutrition in the last few decades is being shown to have been based on faulty premises, and that it's stubborn persistence deserves to be taken about as seriously as the plot of a *Seinfeld* episode.

Know your badditives and how to avoid them:

PARTIALLY HYDROGENATED OILS (TRANS FATS)

- While the FDA says that PHOs, which are the source of trans fats, will be out of the food supply by mid-June of 2018, numerous foods containing them will remain on supermarket shelves for at least eighteen months, and quite likely longer. So continue to watch out for any and all partially hydrogenated oils in processed foods.
- Don't rely on the Nutrition Facts label statement of "no trans fats." Because of a long-standing FDA loophole, amounts less than 0.5 grams can be listed as "0."
- Be especially wary of cakes, cookies, crackers, frozen dinners, and ready-to-bake rolls and pizza crust, as well as some solid shortenings sold for baking, which are the most likely places that you'll find PHOs.

rBGH or rBST

The Banished Badditive That Never Quite Went Away

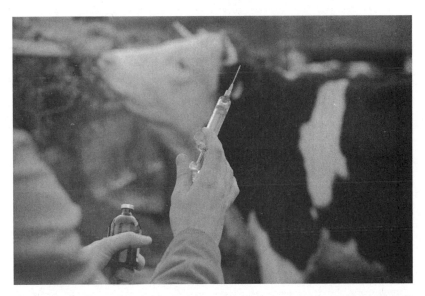

Credit: iStock

"As scientists and consumer advocates warned at the start, revving up cows with a powerful synthetic hormone for no other reason than to force them to produce about 15 percent more milk is a terrible idea."
—Ronnie Cummins,
Organic Consumers Association

In some respects, the saga of recombinant bovine growth hormone, or rBGH (also known as rBST), appears to be a tale of a Monsanto-made Badditive—the predecessor to those GMOs—that finally got its come-uppance.

This notorious veterinary drug, shot into cows so they will produce greater quantities of milk, looks to have been effectively banished from a large number of American dairy operations. Or has it?

As we found out, that's not always an easy question to get an answer to.

That's because the use of rBGH has never been officially banned in the United States (even though it has in many other countries). Since there's no requirement that its presence be announced, it's not something you can look for on an ingredient label, although you can find dairy products that state they are produced from rBGH-free cows.

Actually, rBGH (or rBST), which is sold under the name Posilac, has the distinction of being the first agricultural product on the market to have been genetically engineered (by inserting the gene responsible for producing it into an *E. coli* bacterium).[259] Like the Roundup Ready seeds that would follow, it was created by Monsanto's biotechnology division as a supposed economic boon to farmers. Its approval by a company-compromised FDA would cause a good deal of dismay throughout scientific circles, perhaps best summed up by the Consumer Policy Institute's Michael Hansen description of it as "the most controversial product ever authorized" by that agency.[260]

A source of potential cancers for consumers and udder troubles for cows

A good summary of the potential health hazards associated with it is provided in a 2007 letter written by two representatives of Oregon Physicians for Social Responsibility (PSR), Chief Scientific Advisor Martin Donohoe and Campaign for Safe Food Project Director Rick North, to the FDA's chief counsel Sheldon T. Bradshaw.

The letter was in response to a complaint made by Monsanto Chief Counsel Brian Lowry that the public was being misled by "no rBGH" claims on dairy product labels, since, in Lowry's view, "milk from cows supplemented with rBST is equivalent in all respects to other milk" (an exact echo of the reasoning the company used to get approval for GMOs).

Lowry's statements, noted Donohoe and North, were ones Oregon PSR both strongly disagreed with and disputed the accuracy of.

For example, the pair referred to Lowry's assertion that "milk from cows supplemented with rBST is equivalent in all respects to other milk" as "incorrect."

"As Dr. Michael Hansen of Consumers Union pointed out, Monsanto's Posilac adds one amino acid (methionine) to the cow's natural growth hormone molecule. It has been demonstrated that even small differences in this molecular structure can significantly change immunogenic properties. Therefore, rBGH is different than the cow's natural BGH and can be detected by the immune system," they wrote.

What most concerned them, however, was the likelihood that adding rBGH to milk significantly escalated the amounts of another hormone, insulin-like growth factor-1 (IGF-1). As their letter stated, "both laboratory and epidemiological studies have demonstrated that elevated levels of IGF-1 are associated with increases in several types of cancer in humans," including breast, prostate, and colon cancer. One such study, they pointed out, showed that men with higher levels of IGF-1 were four times likelier to develop prostate cancer than those with lower levels. And while IGF-1 in milk "was originally thought to be destroyed by digestion, unable to reach the bloodstream where it could affect cancer rates," studies conducted after 1993 "indicate that casein, the main protein in milk, protects most IGF-1 from digestion."

Donohoe and North also replied to Lowry's claim that "the use of rBST has no harmful effects on cows" by pointing out that "Monsanto's own package insert for Posilac® lists 16 different harmful conditions that this drug increases in cows," including mastitis, a painful udder infection (and a source of pus in milk) treated with antibiotics such as penicillin, amoxicillin, and erythromycin. "Bacteria resistant to these antibiotics are selected out and end up in the milk, air, soil, and water, which can contribute to increased antibiotic resistance in humans," they asserted.

The pair added that the agency's decision to approve rBGH had drawn "widespread criticism from government leaders, farmers, and numerous scientists," including several within the FDA itself. In addition to human health concerns, the governments of Canada and all twenty-five nations of the European Union formally cite physical harm to cows as justification for their banning of rBGH.[261] (It's also been banned in Japan, Australia, New Zealand, and Israel.[262])

As for Lowry's claim that the public was being misled, they noted that Lowry himself had admitted most companies were using the disclaimer included in FDA guidelines, which states that "no significant difference" exists between rBGH and rBGH-free milk.

Donohoe and North also urged that labeling restrictions not be placed on dairy products, noting how "knowledge about the science-based concerns with rBGH is rapidly spreading and consumers are increasingly 'voting with their dollars'"—something they pointed out was "not lost on business leaders, who are making perfectly logical decisions to discontinue rBGH to preserve and enhance their profits." In closing, they recommended that "based on a significant body of scientific research conducted since 1993," rBGH be removed from the market immediately.[263]

Obviously, however, that last bit of advice wasn't heeded. As a result, this secret ingredient that's been nearly forgotten about might still be present in various dairy products, ranging from cheese to ice cream, unless their labels specify otherwise. And the labels that do so have been a huge bone of contention between Monsanto and many dairy companies and co-ops, with the FDA squarely in the middle of the squabble.

A campaign to curtail labeling and suppress information

Originally submitted to the FDA in 1987, rBGH wasn't given an official stamp of approval until six years later while former Monsanto counsel and future vice president Michael Taylor was serving as deputy commissioner for policy there, during which he also approved the first transgenic Monsanto seeds. (For the record, Taylor, whose career has been a flagrant example of the "revolving door" between private corporations and regulatory agencies, has since returned as deputy commissioner for foods under the Obama administration).

The FDA approval was one based on two rat studies submitted by Monsanto, one that lasted four weeks and the second three months, in which the animals were fed rBGH to see if it affected their gastrointestinal systems. In both cases, it was said to have had no effect, a conclusion that Dr. Hansen has disputed.

Contrary to the agency's claims, Hansen told author and activist Marie-Monique Robin (as noted in her book, *The World According to Monsanto*) that antibodies were produced in 20 to 30 percent of the rats studied, meaning "their immune systems had been mobilized to detect and neutralize pathogenic agents." He also charged that the publication of an article on the subject, written by two FDA scientists in the journal *Science*, was "pure and simple manipulation," especially since it was peer-reviewed by a Cornell professor whom Monsanto had paid to test rBGH on cows.[264]

The purpose of injecting dairy cows with rBGH on a twice-monthly schedule was to increase their output of milk by 15 percent[265]—which at the time it was introduced was uncalled-for at best since the market was already glutted with milk.[266] While it may have temporarily boosted the bottom lines of some dairy farmers (along with Monsanto's), the use of rBGH also raised fears among leading scientists and watchdog groups that it was subjecting Americans to some new and wholly unnecessary risks, especially given that children are the prime consumers of milk in this country. As consumer advocate and author Robyn O'Brien pointed out in a 2015 blog, a recent study published in the *Journal of Allergy and Immunology* found that milk is now the most common food allergy trigger in the US, having achieved that distinction in the last decade.[267] Coincidence?

Such concerns were heightened by the FDA's stated refusal to require that products containing rBGH be specially labeled or that distributors be informed of its presence. All this because, of course, the agency had declared it as having no effect on the quality of milk.

Fortunately, in this case, a campaign waged by activists and whistleblowers to create public awareness of these hazards proved effective enough to encourage quite a few commercial dairies and co-ops to go rBGH-free. Many of their milk suppliers weren't inclined to put up much resistance in any event, given the economic problems it was causing them, such as having to take sick cows out of production and give them antibiotics to treat mastitis, as well as being offered less money for their milk due to its having to be segregated.[268]

As far as the FDA is concerned, however, there's been no cause to revisit that initial approval. While the agency did allow dairies to let consumers know when their products came from cows that had not been treated with the hormone, its guidelines recommended that any such labeling include a disclaimer that "no significant difference has been shown between milk derived from rBST-treated and non-rBST-treated cows." That disclaimer, according to Robin, was signed by Taylor in 1994, but was actually drafted by yet another former Monsanto employee, Dr. Margaret Miller, then deputy director at the FDA's Center for Veterinary Medicine (something the author claims Taylor verbally acknowledged to her).[269]

Monsanto, however, wasn't satisfied. It urged the FDA to take much stronger action by sending out warning letters to rBST-free dairy producers, stating that "it is in the public's interest that such (labeling) practices be confronted, addressed, and stopped," as well as asking the Federal Trade Commission to investigate advertising with a similar purpose.[270]

When the FDA proved unwilling to comply, Monsanto sought to have such restraints issued on a state-by-state level. In Ohio, for example, the state Department of Agriculture in 2008 adopted a regulation prohibiting the labeling of milk from non-rBGH-treated cows as "false and misleading," only to have it overturned by the Sixth Circuit Court, which ruled there was some difference after all between milk from treated and untreated cows (and that Ohio's ban on using an asterisk to denote the latter was in violation of the First Amendment.)[271]

Another such labeling ban ordered by the Pennsylvania Department of Agriculture was blocked by then Governor Ed Rendell after drawing protests from consumers. A similar ban passed by the Kansas Legislature in 2009 was vetoed by Governor Kathleen Sibelius.[272] (Interestingly enough, Monsanto has recently found itself in a position of challenging rather than courting state governments, such as Vermont's, for requiring that GMOs in processed foods be labeled.)

The company, however, went even further, using its extensive legal resources to file lawsuits against a number of dairy enterprises for letting their customers know rBGH was *verboten* in their operations, apparently hoping to discourage others in the industry from doing likewise. At first this tactic succeeded in making a few companies back down, but in 2003, in a well-publicized case, the Oakhurst Dairy of Maine, whose rBGH-free claim was actively supported by state officials, refused, eventually agreeing in a settlement only to add the FDA disclaimer to its label.

Another Monsanto attempt at censorship—one that initially succeeded in putting the kibosh on a television news exposé of problems associated with rBGH—resulted in what has since become a somewhat legendary legal battle that ended up putting the issue in the very spotlight the company had hoped to avoid (see box).

Ultimately, such relentless suppression strategies failed to succeed in stemming a steady drop in sales for a synthetic growth hormone that had once been expected by some economists to capture between 63 and 98 percent of the market. Its sharp decline in popularity among dairy farmers was reflected in a study drawn from USDA survey data, which found that its overall use had fallen by two-thirds and that customers whose herds number over a thousand cows had dropped from an estimated 44 percent of such operations in 2005 to just 16 percent in 2010.[273] By 2014, according to the most recent data for dairies from the National Animal Health Monitoring System surveys, only 9.7 percent of dairy operations reported using rBGH with roughly 14.7 percent of dairy cows still being injected with it.[274]

The Monsanto censorship attempt that backfired, big time

The old adage that "knowledge is power" has never been better illustrated than in the way a little knowledge has empowered consumers to convince many dairy companies and cooperatives to keep rBGH out of their products. Perhaps that accounts for the legal intimidation tactics that have been used to keep such knowledge from being disseminated to the public.

A case in point is what happened to an award-winning husband-and-wife investigative reporting team who looked into the controversy surrounding the use of rBGH two decades ago for a television station in Tampa, Florida, only to have the plug pulled on their much-anticipated four-part report at the last minute.

The duo, Jane Akre and Steve Wilson, who had been extensively hyped by Channel 13 as "the Investigators" who "uncover the truth" and "protect you," were planning to reveal how rBGH was approved without its effects on children and adults who drank the resulting milk being adequately tested, and to talk about the studies that linked its use to cancer in humans. However, after Fox News, which had just purchased the outlet, was threatened in a letter from a high-powered Monsanto attorney with "dire consequences" if the report was aired, the station abruptly cancelled the broadcast.[275]

In an attempt to reach an accommodation with Fox attorneys, Akre and Wilson subsequently attempted to revamp the report a total of 83 times, but to no avail, and then were offered a payoff to keep quiet and forget about the whole affair. Finally, they were terminated in December 1997. They subsequently filed a lawsuit claiming they were dismissed "without cause" after refusing to participate in a deliberate misrepresentation of the news, which violated a newly passed Florida whistleblower law.

A jury ended up awarding Akre $425,000, but it was eventually overturned by a state appeals court on the rather cynical premise that lying to the public was not anything a media company was prohibited from doing under the law. (That might also have obligated them to reimburse Fox for $2 million in legal expenses, had not the Florida Supreme Court spared them that indignity.) In 2007, the FCC denied their challenge to the station's license.

Despite those legal defeats and having their case perhaps understandably shunned by other media, the two intrepid journalists became the recipients of various honors that included the 2001 Goldman Environmental Prize for North America, as well as the Joe Callaway Award for Civic Courage, the First Amendment Award of the Society of Professional Journalists, and a special Alliance for Democracy award for Heroism in Journalism.[276] They were also featured in a 2003 documentary, *The Corporation*, which dealt with the details of the whistleblower suit they had initiated, which was also named as "one of the most censored stories" of that year by Project Censored.

All that recognition was no doubt a contributing factor in making people aware of what was secretly being added to the dairy products they and their kids were consuming on a daily basis—and in the subsequent decision of so many dairy farms to get rid of it.

Still a shadowy presence

That downward trend, no doubt, was helped along by a number of retail bans on milk and dairy products from hormone-treated cows. Among the organizations excluding their use were major chains like Kroger, Safeway, and Walmart, whose store brands became rBGH-free, as well as various makers of nonorganic dairy products, such as Breyers and Ben & Jerry's ice cream and Cabot Creamery Cooperative, a producer of cheese owned by farmers in New England and New York. According to Communications Director Doug Dimento, Cabot's board of directors notified the cooperative's members that as of January 2016, they must either refrain from any further use of the drug or find another market for their products. After having already advised them five years previously that "our customers don't want rBST," he added, it was determined that no more than 2 percent were still using it. (Despite that, Dimento was careful to note, Cabot can't absolutely guarantee that its aged cheese products might not have come from treated cows.)

While Dimento frankly acknowledged that Cabot's ban on the artificial growth hormone was in direct response to the concerns expressed by consumers, it hasn't yet moved the entire cheese industry to reject it. In surveying some other producers, we were told by a consumer affairs representative for Sargento that the Wisconsin-based "natural cheese" company simply urges its suppliers to avoid rBGH. A call to the consumer hotline of one of the country's biggest cheese manufacturers, Kraft Foods, revealed that the corporation doesn't appear to be at all concerned about the issue. "We are not rejecting milk from rBST- and rBGH-supplemented herds," we were informed by a spokesman, who indicated that Kraft was relying on the FDA's having "assured" that it was identical to milk from nonsupplemented cows.

The good news, however, is that unlike GMOs, were its use to be ended completely, there would be no lasting effect on the food supply, according to North.

Eventually, the combination of controversy, corporate boycotts, and slumping sales may have proven too much even for Monsanto, which, having switched its main focus by then to the widespread marketing of

Roundup Ready transgenic seeds, sold the entire division responsible for rBGH to the pharmaceutical firm Eli Lilly in 2008.[277]

Just as in other instances cited in this book, the failure of the FDA to reconsider a previous approval, despite evidence that increasingly contradicts its advisability, continues to create lingering doubts about the safety of far too many products on the shelves of our supermarkets that needn't have ever been a source of concern to us.

The widespread public rejection of rBGH was no doubt a model for Monsanto showing what the "right to know" can do to profitability—one that may well have influenced it to spend millions of dollars fighting GMO labeling initiatives. Its shameless attempts to keep the public totally in the dark about whether or not products may harbor a potentially dangerous drug should, in turn, serve as a constant reminder to consumers of the lengths to which some enterprises will go to milk any method to get extra revenues, no matter what the consequences for society.

Know your badditives and how to avoid them:

rBGH or rBST

- Unless you're buying all organic milk and dairy, check to see if the label contains a notice that the product is supposed to be rBHG-free. Some companies state that they only purchase milk from farms that don't use it. For example, Ben & Jerry's labels state: "The family farmers who supply our milk and cream pledge not to treat their cows with rBGH." (While such a "pledge" isn't a guarantee, it's more likely than not to be honored if a reputable company is involved.)
- You might also try products made from goat's milk. While goats can also be given rBHG, it's much less likely. Goat farms are still typically small family operations. You can buy organic goat's milk, yogurt, and cheese as well.

A WRAP-UP

Recapping the thirteen *baddest* badditives—and why you should avoid them

ALUMINUM: This common metal, compounds of which are added to many processed foods from cake mixes to frozen fish (as well as to antacids, antiperspirants, and cosmetics) for a whole variety of reasons, has now been directly linked to the development of Alzheimer's disease. In addition, recent research has suggested it may be a risk factor for inflammatory bowel diseases.

ARTIFICIAL COLORS: These petroleum-based food dyes, long used to make snack foods and other processed products look more appealing, have been identified by researchers as a likely cause of hyperactivity and learning problems in the classroom. In fact, the Feingold Association of the United States has successfully treated many kids with ADHD by systematically removing foods containing such coloring agents from their diets.

ASPARTAME: Hyped as a "healthy" sugar substitute, this no-calorie synthetic sweetener has actually been linked to a long list of adverse reactions (including obesity). It is also classified as an "excitotoxin," a type of neurotransmitter that can kill certain brain cells when consumed by children and neurologically vulnerable older people.

BHA, BHT (Butylated hydroxyanisole, butylated hydroxytoluene): Like artificial colors, these petroleum-based preservatives have been identified as probable perpetrators of the ADHD epidemic that often results in kids being put on risky drugs. Researchers have also found evidence that implicates both as likely suspects in the development of certain cancers and other health problems.

CARRAGEENAN: Used as a thickener, this seaweed derivative, which, by virtue of being "natural," is even allowed in organic foods, has been implicated by a sizable body of research as a cause of gastrointestinal problems that can result in serious illness.

FLUORIDE: This toxic chemical, which can easily find its way into your food from the water you cook with or that has been used in food processing, is actually an industrial waste product deliberately added to drinking water as a tooth decay preventive. Many scientists, however, including some veterans of the EPA, warn that it can be hazardous to your family's health—as well as to their teeth. And the real reasons it's in the water in the first place may make you cringe.

GMOs (genetically modified organisms): Allowed on the market without the benefit of any safety testing whatsoever, the transgenic ingredients now found in the great majority of nonorganic processed foods pose potentially disastrous long-term health, allergy, and environmental risks—as does the glyphosate herbicide most of them were created to accommodate.

HIGH FRUCTOSE CORN SYRUP (HFCS): This laboratory-synthesized sweetener, used as a cheap substitute for sugar in a wide variety of processed foods, has been identified by researchers as a major contributor to the current epidemics of obesity and diabetes, as well as being linked to heart ailments, nonalcoholic fatty liver disease, pancreatic cancer, asthma, and cognition problems.

MEAT GLUE: Though eclipsed by the revulsion over so-called "pink slime," this bacteria-generated enzyme, technically known as transglutaminase, can be far more of a health hazard. Used to make fake steak, fish filets, and other deceiving dishes from meat, seafood, or poultry scraps, it can provide a pathway for pathogens that can really make you sick; and it could set the stage for some serious chronic diseases as well.

MSG AND ITS VARIOUS DISGUISES: Despite industry and government assurances that they're nothing much to worry about, monosodium glutamate and related forms of free glutamic acid, such as hydrolyzed protein, sodium caseinate, and autolyzed yeast (all of which can be referred to as "MSG"), have a long history of producing adverse effects, which in especially sensitive individuals can be serious and even life-threatening. Like aspartame, free glutamate is also an "excitotoxin" that can "zap" certain brain cells in children and older people.

PARTIALLY HYDROGENATED OILS (PHOs): Used to give processed foods a longer shelf life, these sources of artery-clogging trans fats have been blamed for shortening the lives of thousands of American consumers. In fact, they cause about seven thousand heart disease–related deaths a year, according to an estimate by the FDA, which has belatedly been pressured into phasing them out—although it may take a while before they're no longer listed as an ingredient in numerous products.

rBGH OR rBST (recombinant bovine growth hormone): This genetically engineered growth hormone, injected into dairy herds to make them produce more milk, has been linked to both cancer in humans and health problems in cows that have resulted in an increased use of antibiotics. But while its use has been significantly reduced as a result, it's still allowed and can still be found in dairy products that aren't organic or labeled as non-rBGH.

By reducing or eliminating your family's consumption of foods containing these pernicious substances, you'll not only be helping yourself and your children to steer clear of the various afflictions that plague our society, from diabetes and heart disease to cancer and Alzheimer's, but also giving food manufacturers one more reason to stop using them.

By spreading the word about these badditives to your relatives, friends, and neighbors, you can become part of the resistance movement now well on its way to reforming an industry that has been allowed to compromise the health and well-being of the American public for far too long.

REFERENCES

ALUMINUM

1. Robert A. Yokel, "Aluminum in Food: The Nature and Contribution of Food Additives," in *Food Additive*, ed. Yehia El-Samragy (InTech, 2012) p. 206, http://cdn.intechopen.com/pdfs-wm/28917.pdf.
2. Ibid, p. 205.
3. Ibid, pp. 205–206.
4. A. Khalil Enas, "Study the Possible Protective and Therapeutic Influence of Coriander (Coriandrum sativum L.) Against Neurodegenerative Disorders and Alzheimer's disease Induced by Aluminum Chloride in Cerebral Cortex of Male Albino Rats," *Nature and Science*, 2010, http://www.sciencepub.net/nature/ns0811/27_4062ns0811_202_213.pdf.
5. Keele University, "Early onset Alzheimer's disease in worker exposed to aluminium," 2014, http://www.keele.ac.uk/pressreleases/2014/earlyonsetalzheimersdiseaseinworkerexposedtoaluminium.html.
6. Future Science, "The first clinical trial testing the link between Alzheimer's disease and Aluminium," 2015, https://www.futsci.com/project/the-aluminium-alzheimer-s-disease-hypothesis-what-is-the-role-of-aluminium-in-alzheimers-disease.
7. Keele University, "Early onset Alzheimer's disease in worker exposed to aluminium," 2014, http://www.keele.ac.uk/pressreleases/2014/earlyonsetalzheimersdiseaseinworkerexposedtoaluminium.html.
8. Future Science, "The first clinical trial testing the link between Alzheimer's disease and Aluminium," 2014, https://www.futsci.com/project/the-aluminium-alzheimer-s-disease-hypothesis-what-is-the-role-of-aluminium-in-alzheimers-disease.
9. Christopher Exley, "Why industry propaganda and political interference cannot disguise the inevitable role played by human exposure to aluminum in neurodegenerative diseases, including Alzheimer's disease," *Frontiers in Neurology*, October 2014, p. 212, http://journal.frontiersin.org/article/10.3389/fneur.2014.00212/full.

10. Keele University, "Early onset Alzheimer's disease in worker exposed to aluminium," 2014, http://www.keele.ac.uk/pressreleases/2014/earlyonsetalzheimersdiseaseinworkerexposedtoaluminium.html.

11. Christopher Exley, "Why industry propaganda and political interference cannot disguise the inevitable role played by human exposure to aluminum in neurodegenerative diseases, including Alzheimer's disease," *Frontiers in Neurology*, October 2014, p. 212, http://journal.frontiersin.org/article/10.3389/fneur.2014.00212/full.

12. Chia-Yi Yuan et al., "Aluminum overload increases oxidative stress in four functional brain areas of neonatal rats," Journal of Biomedical Science, May 2012, http://www.ncbi.nlm.nih.gov/pmc/articles/PMC3404950/.

13. Keele University, "Early onset Alzheimer's disease in worker exposed to aluminium," 2014, http://www.keele.ac.uk/pressreleases/2014/earlyonsetalzheimersdiseaseinworkerexposedtoaluminium.html.

14. C. Vignal et al., "Gut: An underestimated target organ for Aluminum," *Morphologie*, March 2016, http://www.sciencedirect.com/science/article/pii/S1286011516000266.

15. R. Keith McCormick, *The Whole-Body Approach to Osteoporosis* (Vancouver: Raincoast Books, 2009), p. 150.

ARTIFICIAL COLORS

16. Allan Magaziner, Linda Bonvie, and Anthony Zolezzi, *Chemical-Free Kids* (New York: Twin Streams, 2003), p. 40.

17. Michael Greger, "Red Dye No. 3 and Thyroid Cancer," 2015, http://nutritionfacts.org/2015/04/30/coloring-to-dye-for-dangers-of-red-no-3/.

18. Michael Greger, "Red Dye No. 3 and Thyroid Cancer," 2015, http://nutritionfacts.org/2015/04/30/coloring-to-dye-for-dangers-of-red-no-3/.

19. Oliver Nieburg, "Hershey's Milk Chocolate and Kisses to go non-GM," 2015, http://www.confectionerynews.com/Ingredients/Hershey-in-non-GMO-and-no-high-fructose-corn-syrup-pledge.

20. Mars, Incorporated, "Mars, Incorporated to remove all artificial colors from its human food portfolio," 2016, http://www.prnewswire.com/news-releases/mars-incorporated-to-remove-all-artificial-colors-from-its-human-food-portfolio-300216158.html.

21. Katie Bratskeir, "11 Companies that Plan to Remove Artificial Flavors By 2018," *The Huffington Post*, 2015, http://www.huffingtonpost.com/entry/11-companies-that-plan-to-remove-artificial-flavors-before-2019_us_55b6a777e4b0074ba5a5d327.

22. Center for Science in the Public Interest, "CSPI Urges FDA to Ban Artificial Food Dyes Linked to Behavior Problems," 2008, http://www.cspinet.org/new/200806022.html.

23. US Food and Drug Administration, "Quick Minutes: Food Advisory Committee Meeting March 30-31, 2011," 2011, http://www.fda.gov/AdvisoryCommittees/CommitteesMeetingMaterials/FoodAdvisoryCommittee/ucm250901.htm.

24. Richard W. Pressinger, Chem-tox.com, "Food Colorings Given Following Birth Generate Attention Deficit Disorder Symptoms," 1997, http://www.chem-tox.com/pregnancy/artificial.htm.

25. Donna McCann, "Food additives and hyperactive behaviour in 3-year-old and 8/9-year-old children in the community: a randomised, double-blinded, placebo-controlled trial," *The Lancet*, 2007, http://www.feingold.org/Research/PDFstudies/Stevenson2007.pdf, p. 7.

26. The Feingold Association of the United States, "American Academy of Pediatrics ADHD and Food Additives Revisited," 2008, http://www.feingold.org/aap.html.

27. Center for Science in the Public Interest, "The Science Linking Food dyes with Impacts on Children's Behavior, CSPI," 2016, https://www.cspinet.org/fooddyes/Food-Dyes-Fact-Sheet.pdf.

28. Ibid.

29. Laurel Curran, "EU Places Warning Labels on Foods Containing Dyes," 2010, http://www.foodsafetynews.com/2010/07/eu-places-warning-labels-on-foods-containing-dyes/#.V05ZbY-cHm.

30. Allergysymptomsx.com, "Red Dye Allergy," http://allergysymptomsx.com/red-dye-allergy.php.

31. Kirsten Fischer, "Is Red Dye 40 Toxic?," 2015, http://www.healthline.com/health/food-nutrition/is-red-dye-40-toxic.

32. Elaine Watson, "LycoRed reports rocketing demand for lycopene-based red color as firms seek alternatives to carmine," 2012, http://www.foodnavigator-usa.com/Markets/LycoRed-reports-rocketing-demand-for-lycopene-based-red-color-as-firms-seek-alternatives-to-carmine.

33. Tammy Dray, "Health Effects of Yellow 5 Food Coloring," 2015, http://www.livestrong.com/article/370945-health-effects-of-yellow-5-food-coloring/.

34. The Alternative Daily, "Top 5 Worst Artificial Colors," http://www.thealternativedaily.com/top-5-worst-artificial-colors/.

35. Michelle Kmiec, "Food Dyes & Additives Proven Unsafe!," 2015, http://www.onlineholistichealth.com/food-dyes-additives-proven-unsafe/.

36. The Feingold Association of the United States, *The Feingold Bluebook*, 2012, http://www.feingold.org/BLUEBOOK.pdf.

37. Center for Science in the Public Interest, "Food Dyes: A Rainbow of Risks," 2010, https://cspinet.org/new/pdf/food-dyes-rainbow-of-risks.pdf.

38. Uncle Wiley's, "The Color of Health", https://unclewileys.com/index.php/content/view/42/40/.

ASPARTAME

39. National PKU Alliance, "About PKU," 2014, http://npkua.org/Education/About-PKU.
40. United States Food and Drug Administration, "Additional Information about High-Intensity Sweeteners Permitted for use in Food in the United States," 2015, http://www.fda.gov/Food/IngredientsPackagingLabeling/FoodAdditivesIngredients/ucm397725.htm.
41. Phone interview with Mary Nash Stoddard.
42. Email to the authors from Mark Gold.
43. Linda and Bill Bonvie, "Sinfully Sweet," *New Age Journal*, February 1996, p. 126.
44. United States Food and Drug Administration, "Reported Aspartame Toxicity Effects," 2003, http://www.fda.gov/ohrms/dockets/dailys/03/jan03/012203/02p-0317_emc-000199.txt.
45. Blaylock, Russel, *Excitotoxins: the Taste that Kills* (Santa Fe: Health Press, 1994), pp. 194–195.
46. Arthur M. Evangelista, "Aspartame: The History Of A Killer—The Whole Story," http://www.rense.com/general50/killer.htm.
47. Ibid.
48. Rich Murray, "How Aspartame Became Legal—the Timeline," http://www.rense.com/general33/legal.htm.
49. Ibid.
50. Marie-Monique Robin, *Our Daily Poison* (New York: The New Press, 2014), p. 271.
51. Rich Murray, "How Aspartame Became Legal—The Timeline," http://www.rense.com/general33/legal.htm.
52. MD Health, "What Foods Contain Aspartame?," http://www.md-health.com/What-Foods-Contain-Aspartame.html.
53. Linda Bonvie, "An interview with Citizens for Health Board Chair James S. Turner," 2014, http://foodidentitytheft.com/an-interview-with-citizens-for-health-board-chair-james-s-turner/.
54. Robin, op. cit, p. 272.
55. Robin, op. cit, p. 271.
56. Howard M. Metzenbaum, "Metzenbaum Questions Hatch: Letter to Senator Hatch, Feb 3," 2016, http://dorway.com/history-of-aspartame/how-did-aspartame-get-approved-by-the-fda/dead-bill/letter-to-hatch-feb-3/.
57. Ellen Ruppel Shell, "Artificial Sweeteners May Change Our Gut Bacteria in Dangerous Ways," 2015, http://www.scientificamerican.com/article/artificial-sweeteners-may-change-our-gut-bacteria-in-dangerous-ways/.

58. University of Manitoba News, "Artificially sweetened beverages consumed in pregnancy linked to increased weight gain in infants," 2016, http://news.umanitoba.ca/artificially-sweetened-beverages-consumed-in-pregnancy-linked-to-increased-weight-gain-in-infants/.

59. Blaylock, op. cit., pp. 211–213.

60. Ibid.

61. Betty Martini, "Report for Schools, OB-GYN and Pediatricians on Children and Aspartame/MSG," 2016, http://www.mpwhi.com/report_on_aspartame_and_children.htm.

62. Blaylock, op. cit., pp. 211–213.

63. Our Alexander "Increase in Pediatric Brain Tumors," http://www.ouralexander.org/increase.htm.

64. Center for Science in the Public Interest, "Taylor Swift Urged to 'Shake Off' Aspartame," 2015, http://www.cspinet.org/new/201501161.html.

65. University of Iowa Health Care Marketing and Communications, "UI study finds diet drinks associated with heart trouble for older women," 2014, http://now.uiowa.edu/2014/03/ui-study-finds-diet-drinks-associated-heart-trouble-older-women.

66. Glenda Lindseth et al., "Neurobehavioral effects of aspartame consumption," *Research in Nursing & Health*, June 2014, http://www.ncbi.nlm.nih.gov/pubmed/24700203.

67. Calorie Control Council, "Aspartame Myths," http://www.aspartame.org/myths-facts/aspartame-myths/.

68. Ken Stoller, "Santa Fe Pediatrician Ken Stoller Asks FDA to Rescind Aspartame's Approval," 2009, http://www.opednews.com/articles/2/Santa-Fe-Pediatrician-Ken-by-Ken-Stoller-M-D-090918-695.html.

69. Steven Musser, "Citizen Petition Denial Letter Response from FDA CFSAN to Paul Stoller MD," 2014, https://www.regulations.gov/document?D=FDA-2009-P-0156-0003.

70. Steven Musser, "Citizen Petition Denial Letter Response from FDA CFSAN to Betty Martini," 2014, https://www.regulations.gov/document?D=FDA-2002-P-0247-0023.

71. H. J. Roberts, *Aspartame Disease: An Ignored Epidemic* (West Palm Beach: Sunshine Sentinel Press, 2001), p. 5.

72. Mission Possible World Health International, "Pilot Aspartame Alert," 2011, http://www.mpwhi.com/pilot_aspartame_alert_with_letters.htm, interview by co-author Bill Bonvie.

73. Ibid.

74. "Aspartame Alert," US Air Force, *Flying Safety*, May, 1992, pp. 20, 21.

75. "Mail Call," US Air Force, *Flying Safety*, August, 1992, p. 13.

76. Linda and Bill Bonvie, "Sinfully Sweet?," *New Age Journal*, February 1996, p. 60.

77. Kaitlin M. Baudier et al., "Erythritol, a Non-Nutritive Sugar Alcohol Sweetener and the Main Component of Truvia®, Is a Palatable Ingested Insecticide," *PLOS ONE*, June 2014, http://journals.plos.org/plosone/article?id=10.1371/journal.pone.0098949.

BHA and BHT

78. The Feingold Association of the United States, "Let's Not Forget the BHT, BHA & TBHQ," http://www.feingold.org/enews/03-2010.html.
79. The Feingold Association of the United States, "Preservatives," http://feingold.org/about-the-program/what-is-the-feingold-program/preservatives/.
80. Phone interview with Jane Hersey by Bill Bonvie.
81. John D. Stokes and Charles L. Scudder, "The effect of butylated hydroxyanisole and butylated hydroxytoluene on behavioral development of mice, "*Developmental Psychobiology*, July 1974, 343–350, https://www.ncbi.nlm.nih.gov/pubmed/4472726.
82. The Feingold Association of the United States, *The Feingold Bluebook*, 2012, http://www.feingold.org/DOCS/Bluebook-phone.pdf, p. 44.
83. J. A. Thompson et al., "A metabolite of butylated hydroxytoluene with potent tumor-promoting activity in mouse lung." *Carcinogenesis*, April 1989, http://www.ncbi.nlm.nih.gov/pubmed/2702725.
84. Ibid, p. 46.
85. Scorecard, "Known Carcinogens and Reproductive Toxicants (California Proposition 65)," http://scorecard.goodguide.com/chemical-groups/one-list.tcl?short_list_name=p65.
86. The Endocrine Disruption Exchange, "Endocrine Disruption TEDX List of Potential Endocrine Disruptors," http://endocrinedisruption.org/popup-chemical-details?chemid=907.
87. P. J. Hughes et al., "Estrogenic alkylphenols induce cell death by inhibiting testis endoplasmic reticulum Ca(2+) pumps." *Biochemical and Biophysical Research Communications*, September 2000, http://www.ncbi.nlm.nih.gov/pubmed/11061995.
88. Geri Kelley and Sarina Gleason, "Common Additive May Be Why You Have Food Allergies," 2016, http://msutoday.msu.edu/news/2016/common-additive-may-be-why-you-have-food-allergies/.
89. Food Babe, "Kellogg's & General Mills: Drop the BHT From Your Cereal – Like You Do In Other Countries!" http://foodbabe.com/cereal/.
90. Elaine Watson, "Gen Mills 'well down path' of removing BHT from cereals; Kellogg 'actively testing natural alternatives,'" 2015, http://www.foodnavigator-usa.com/Manufacturers/Gen-Mills-Kellogg-under-fire-from-Food-Babe-over-BHT-in-cereals.

CARRAGEENAN

91. The Cornucopia Institute, "Carrageenan: New Studies Reinforce Link to Inflammation, Cancer and Diabetes," 2016, p. 18, http://www.cornucopia.org/wp-content/uploads/2016/04/CarageenanReport-2016.pdf.

92. The Cornucopia Institute, "Carrageenan: New Studies Reinforce Link to Inflammation, Cancer and Diabetes," 2013, p. 7, http://www.cornucopia.org/wp-content/uploads/2013/02/Carrageenan-Report1.pdf.

93. The Cornucopia Institute, "Carrageenan: New Studies Reinforce Link to Inflammation, Cancer and Diabetes," 2013, http://www.cornucopia.org/wp-content/uploads/2013/03/Cornucopia-Carrageenan-Petition-3-15-2013.pdf.

94. The Cornucopia Institute, "Carrageenan: New Studies Reinforce Link to Inflammation, Cancer and Diabetes," 2013, pp. 11–12, http://www.cornucopia.org/wp-content/uploads/2013/02/Carrageenan-Report1.pdf.

95. The Cornucopia Institute, "Carrageenan: New Studies Reinforce Link to Inflammation, Cancer and Diabetes," 2013, pp. 11–12, http://www.cornucopia.org/wp-content/uploads/2013/02/Carrageenan-Report1.pdf.

96. The Cornucopia Institute, "Carrageenan: New Studies Reinforce Link to Inflammation, Cancer and Diabetes," 2016, pp. 18, 22, http://www.cornucopia.org/wp-content/uploads/2016/04/CarageenanReport-2016.pdf.

97. Ibid, p. 19.

98. The Cornucopia Institute, "Carrageenan: New Studies Reinforce Link to Inflammation, Cancer and Diabetes," 2016, http://www.cornucopia.org/carrageenan-how-a-natural-food-additive-is-making-us-sick/.

99. Ibid, p. 22.

100. The Cornucopia Institute, "Carrageenan: New Studies Reinforce Link to Inflammation, Cancer and Diabetes," 2016, pp. 13–14, http://www.cornucopia.org/wp-content/uploads/2016/04/CarageenanReport-2016.pdf.

101. The Cornucopia Institute, "Carrageenan: New Studies Reinforce Link to Inflammation, Cancer and Diabetes," 2013, pp. 21–22, http://www.cornucopia.org/wp-content/uploads/2013/02/Carrageenan-Report1.pdf.

102. Food Babe, "Watch Out For This Carcinogen In Your Organic Food," http://foodbabe.com/2012/05/22/watch-out-for-this-carcinogen-in-your-organic-food/.

103. Associated Press, 2014 "WhiteWave to remove ingredient from Horizon, Silk," https://www.yahoo.com/news/whitewave-remove-ingredient-horizon-silk-192520573.html?ref=gs.

FLUORIDE

104. North Carolina Health and Human Services, "Maximum Contaminant Levels (MCLs) for Drinking Water," http://ehs.ncpublichealth.com/oswp/docs/MCL-Handout-2010-01Mar.pdf.

105. Michael Connett, "The Phosphate Fertilizer Industry: An Environmental Overview," 2003, http://fluoridealert.org/articles/phosphate01/.

106. Chris Bryson and Joel Griffiths, "Fluoride, Teeth and the Atomic Bomb," 1997, http://fluoridealert.org/articles/wastenot414/.

107. Ibid.

108. Project Censored, "18. Manhattan Project Covered Up Effects of Fluoride Toxicity," 2010, http://projectcensored.org/18-manhattan-project-covered-up-effects-of-fluoride-toxicity/.

109. American Dental Association, "Fluoridation Facts," 2005, p. 9, http://www.ada.org/~/media/ADA/Member%20Center/FIles/fluoridation_facts.ashx.

110. Chris Bryson and Joel Griffiths, "Fluoride, Teeth and the Atomic Bomb," 1997, http://fluoridealert.org/articles/wastenot414/.

111. Ibid.

112. Toxipedia, "Grand Rapids Fluoridation Trial," 2015, http://www.toxipedia.org/display/toxipedia/Grand+Rapids+Fluoridation+Trial.

113. Christopher Bryson, *The Fluoride Deception*, (New York: Seven Stories Press, 2004), pp. 35–40.

114. Ibid, p. xviii.

115. Ibid, p. 27.

116. Interview with coauthor Bill Bonvie in 2000.

117. New York State Coalition Opposed to Fluoridation, "Fluoridation Increases Lead Absorption in Children," 2000, http://www.lead.org.au/lanv7n4/L74-11.html.

118. Thomas H. Maugh II, "HHS and EPA will recommend lower fluoride levels in water supply," *Los Angeles Times*, January 2011, http://articles.latimes.com/2011/jan/07/news/la-heb-fluoridated-water-0107-2011.

119. Interview with coauthor Bill Bonvie in 2000.

120. María Teresa Alarcón-Herrera et al., "Wellwater Fluoride, Dental Fluorosis, and Bone Fractures in the Guadiana Valley of Mexico," *Fluoride*, 2001, http://www.fluorideresearch.org/342/files/FJ2001_v34_n2_p139-149fig.pdf.

121. Simmi Kharb et al., "Fluoride levels and osteosarcoma," *South Asian Journal of Cancer*, October 2012, http://www.ncbi.nlm.nih.gov/pmc/articles/PMC3876610/.

122. Bryson, op. cit., p. 222.

123. C. Danielson et al., "Hip fractures and fluoridation in Utah's elderly population," *JAMA*, August 1992, http://www.ncbi.nlm.nih.gov/pubmed/1640574.

124. The Fluoride Debate, "DISEASES, Question 30. Does drinking optimally fluoridated water cause or contribute to heart disease," 2001, http://www. fluoridedebate.com/question30.html.

125. Bryson, op. cit., p. 225.

126. Interview with coauthor Bill Bonvie in 2000.

127. Holisticmed.com, "EPA Scientists Take Stand Against Fluoride," http://www. holisticmed.com/fluoride/epa.html.

128. Saundra Young, "Government recommends lowering fluoride levels in U.S. drinking water," CNN, January 2011, http://www.cnn.com/2011/ HEALTH/01/07/fluoride.recommendations/.

129. Fluoridation.com, "Fluoridation status of some countries," http://fluoridation. com/c-country.htm.

130. Fluoridation.com, "Fluoride: Protected Pollutant or Panacea?," http://www. fluoridation.com/.

131. Bryson, op. cit., pp. 227 229.

GMOs

132. Jeffrey M. Smith, *Genetic Roulette* (Fairfield, Iowa: Yes! Books, 2007), p. 176.

133. Ibid, p. 59.

134. Ibid, pp. 32, 38–44, 48.

135. Marta Herbert, "What is Genetically Modified Food (and Why You Should Care)," *EarthSave Magazine*, Spring 2002.

136. Smith, op. cit., p. 51.

137. Ibid, p. 34.

138. Emma Young, "GM pea causes allergic damage in mice," November 2005, https://www.newscientist.com/article/dn8347-gm-pea-causes-allergic-damage-in-mice/.

139. Steven M. Druker, *Altered Genes, Twisted Truths* (Salt Lake City: Clear River Press, 2015), pp. 178–179.

140. Pamela Coleman, "Gut-Wrenching: New Studies Reveal the Insidious Effects of Glyphosate," 2014, http://www.cornucopia.org/2014/03/gut-wrenching-new-studies-reveal-insidious-effects-glyphosate/.

141. Charles M. Benbrook, "Trends in glyphosate herbicide use in the United States and globally," *Environmental Sciences Europe*, February 2016, http://link. springer.com/article/10.1186/s12302-016-0070-0.

142. Zoë Schlanger, "The FDA Will Begin Testing Food for Glyphosate, the Most Heavily Used Farm Chemical Ever," *Newsweek*, February 2016, http://www. newsweek.com/fda-will-begin-testing-food-glyphosate-most-heavily-used-farm-chemical-ever-428790.

143. T. Bøhn et al., "Compositional differences in soybeans on the market: Glyphosate accumulates in Roundup Ready GM soybeans," *Food Chemistry*, June 2014, http://www.sciencedirect.com/science/article/pii/S0308814613019201.

144. Christopher D. Peloso, "Diamond, Commissioner of Patents and Trademarks v. Chakrabarty. U.S. 303 (1980)," http://www.invispress.com/law/property/diamond.html.

145. Rebecca S. Eisenberg, "Story of Diamond v. Chakrabarty, The: Technological Change and the Subject Matter Boundaries of the Patent System," https://www.techpolicy.com/Articles/S/Story-of-Diamond-v-Chakrabarty,-The-Technologica.aspx.

146. United States Department of Agriculture, "Biotechnology Frequently Asked Questions (FAQs)," 2016, http://www.usda.gov/wps/portal/usda/usdahome?navid=AGRICULTURE&contentid=BiotechnologyFAQs.xml.

147. Dave Murphy, "20 years of GMO Policy That Keeps Americans in the Dark About Their Food," *The Huffington Post*, July 2012, http://www.huffingtonpost.com/dave-murphy/dan-quayle-and-michael-ta_b_1551732.html.

148. Ibid.

149. T. Bøhn et al., "Compositional differences in soybeans on the market: Glyphosate accumulates in Roundup Ready GM soybeans," *Food Chemistry*, June 2014, http://www.sciencedirect.com/science/article/pii/S0308814613019201.

150. Druker, op. cit., pp. 1–4.

151. Ibid, p. 131.

152. Ibid, pp. 283–287.

153. Smith, op. cit., pp. 25, 59.

154. Catherine Greene et al., "Economic Issues in the Coexistence of Organic, Genetically Engineered (GE), and Non-GE Crops," February 2016, http://www.ers.usda.gov/publications/eib-economic-information-bulletin/eib-149/report-summary.aspx.

155. Phone interview with Bill Freese, May 2016.

156. Smith, op. cit., p. 7.

157. Bill Freese, "Why GM Crops Will Not Feed the World," in *The GMO Deception* (New York: Skyhorse Publishing, 2014), p. 114.

158. Ibid, p. 113.

159. Kimberly A. C. Wilson, "Genetically engineered sugar beets destroyed in southern Oregon," *The Oregonian*, 2013, http://www.oregonlive.com/pacific-northwest-news/index.ssf/2013/06/genetically_engineered_sugar_b.html.

160. Tamar Haspel, "Scientists Say GMO Foods Are Safe, Public Skepticism Remains," The Plate, 2016, http://theplate.nationalgeographic.com/2016/05/17/scientists-say-gmo-foods-are-safe-public-skepticism-remains/?sf26469099=1.

161. Food & Water Watch, "Under the Influence: The National Research Council and GMOs," 2016, http://www.foodandwaterwatch.org/sites/default/files/ib_1605_nrcinfluence-final-web_0.pdf.

162. Druker, op. cit., p. 402.

163. Ibid, p. 403.

164. Martha L. Crouch, "Patented Seeds vs. Free Inquiry," in *The GMO Deception* (New York: Skyhorse Publishing, 2014).

HIGH FRUCTOSE CORN SYRUP

165. Andrew Weil, "High Fructose Corn Syrup," 2012, https://www.youtube.com/watch?v=FhA6aoKnFCU.

166. Corn Refiners Association, "Sweetners," http://corn.org/products/sweeteners/high-fructose-corn-syrup/.

167. Ibid.

168. Hilary Parker, "A sweet problem: Princeton researchers find that high-fructose corn syrup prompts considerably more weight gain," 2010, http://www.princeton.edu/main/news/archive/S26/91/22K07/.

169. Ibid.

170. Author interview.

171. Corn Refiners Association, "Sweetners," https://web.archive.org/web/20141218173841/http://www.corn.org/products/sweeteners/.

172. Leslie Ridgeway, "High fructose corn syrup linked to diabetes," 2012, https://news.usc.edu/44415/high-fructose corn-syrup-linked-to-diabetes/.

173. Science Daily, "Soda Warning? High-fructose Corn Syrup Linked To Diabetes, New Study Suggests," 2007, http://www.sciencedaily.com/releases/2007/08/070823094819.htm.

174. Al Sears, "HFCS: High Fructose Cancer Syrup," http://www.alsearsmd.com/2014/08/hfcs-high-fructose-cancer-syrup/.

175. Xiaosen Ouyang et al., "Fructose Consumption as a Risk Factor for Non-alcoholic Fatty Liver Disease," *Journal of Hepatology*, June 2008, www.ncbi.nlm.nih.gov/pmc/articles/PMC2423467.

176. Science Daily, "High fructose corn syrup linked to liver scarring, research suggests," March 2010, http://www.sciencedaily.com/releases/2010/03/ 100322204628.htm.

177. Saint Luke's Health System, "Fatty liver disease stronger independent indicator of cardiovascular disease than age, smoking, gender, or other traditional risk factors," 2013, http://www.saintlukeshealthsystem.org/about/news/fatty-liver-disease-stronger-independent-indicator-cardiovascular-disease-age-smoking.

178. Norman K. Pollock et al., "Greater Fructose Consumption Is Associated with Cardiometabolic Risk Markers and Visceral Adiposity in Adolescents," *Journal of Nutrition*, December 2011, http://jn.nutrition.org/content/early/2011/12/20/jn.111.150219.abstract.

179. Science Daily, "Fructose consumption increases risk factors for heart disease: Study suggests US Dietary Guideline for upper limit of sugar consumption is too high," 2011, https://www.sciencedaily.com/releases/2011/07/110728082558.htm.

180. Elaine Schmidt, "This is your brain on sugar: UCLA study shows high-fructose diet sabotages learning, memory," 2012, http://newsroom.ucla.edu/releases/this-is-your-brain-on-sugar-ucla-233992.

181. Elaine Schmidt, "High-fructose diet hampers recovery from traumatic brain injury," 2015, http://newsroom.ucla.edu/releases/high-fructose-diet-hampers-recovery-from-traumatic-brain-injury.

182. Case Adams, "High Fructose Corn Syrup Linked to Asthma and Chronic Bronchitis," http://www.realnatural.org/high-fructose-corn-syrup-linked-to-asthma-and-chronic-bronchitis/.

183. Charles Bankhead, "Mom's, Kid's Fructose Intake Linked to Asthma," 2015, http://www.medpagetoday.com/MeetingCoverage/AAAAI/50205.

184. Case Adams, "High Fructose Corn Syrup Linked to Asthma and Chronic Bronchitis," http://www.realnatural.org/high-fructose-corn-syrup-linked-to-asthma-and-chronic-bronchitis/.

185. Stuart Wolpert, "Fructose alters hundreds of brain genes, which can lead to a wide range of diseases," 2016, http://medicalxpress.com/news/2016-04-fructose-hundreds-brain-genes-wide.html.

186. Ibid.

187. EurekAlert, "Impact of high fructose on health of offspring," 2016, http://www.eurekalert.org/pub_releases/2016-02/sfmm-ioh020416.php.

MEAT GLUE

188. Blanche Levine, "Meat glue found in many common food items," 2012, http://www.naturalhealth365.com/meat-glue.html/.

189. Lily Mihalik, "A Fish Without Bones: The rise of meat glue," June 2011; http://meatpaper.com/articles/2011/mp_fifteen_meatglue.html.

190. Ajinomoto, "Activa TG," http://www.ajiusafood.com/products/enzymes/activa.aspx.

191. Centers for Disease Control and Prevention, "Estimates of Foodborne Illness in the United States," https://www.cdc.gov/foodborneburden.

192. *The Huffington Post*, "In Defense Of Meat Glue," May 2011, http://www.huffingtonpost.com/2011/05/23/defense-meat-glue_n_865545.html.

193. United States Department of Agriculture, "USDA Safety of Transglutaminase Enzyme (TG enzyme)" http://www.fsis.usda.gov/wps/portal/fsis/topics/food-safety-education/get-answers/food-safety-fact-sheets/food-labeling/safety-of-transglutaminase-tg-enzyme/safety-of-tg-enzyme.

194. Federal Register, "Use of Transglutaminase Enzyme and Pork Collagen as Binders in Certain Meat and Poultry Products," October 2001, http://www.fsis.usda.gov/OPPDE/rdad/FRPubs/01-016DF.htm.

195. Federal Register, "Use of Transglutaminase Enzyme and Pork Collagen as Binders in Certain Meat and Poultry Products," March 2002, http://www.fsis.usda.gov/OPPDE/rdad/FRPubs/01-016N.htm.

196. A. Lerner and T. Matthias, "Changes in intestinal tight junction permeability associated with industrial food additives explain the rising incidence of autoimmune disease," *Autoimmunity Reviews*, June 2015, pp. 479–489, https://www.ncbi.nlm.nih.gov/pubmed/25676324.

197. A. Lerner and T. Matthias, "Possible association between celiac disease and bacterial transglutaminase in food processing: a hypothesis," August 2015, http://www.ncbi.nlm.nih.gov/pubmed/26084478.

MSG AND ITS VARIOUS DISGUISES

198. Adreienne Samuels, *The Man Who Sued the FDA*, 2013, pp. 1–3.

199. Ibid, p. 155.

200. Broadwith, Phillip, "Glutamate," Royal Society of Chemistry, June 2011, http://www.rsc.org/images/IC0411-glutamate-food_tcm18-233514.pdf.

201. Samuels, op. cit., pp. 18–19, 84–85.

202. Blaylock, Russell, *Excitotoxins: The Taste That Kills* (Health Press, 1994), p. 55.

203. Samuels, op. cit, p. 95.

204. Ibid.

205. Blaylock, op. cit., p. 56.

206. Ibid, p. 91.

207. Rachel Feltman, "No, MSG isn't bad for you," *Washington Post*, 2014, https://www.washingtonpost.com/news/speaking-of-science/wp/2014/08/25/no-msg-isnt-bad-for-you/.

208. American Chemical Society, "Committee on Corporation Associates," https://www.acs.org/content/acs/en/about/governance/committees/associates.html.

209. US National Library of Medicine, "Chinese restaurant syndrome," https://www.nlm.nih.gov/medlineplus/ency/article/001126.htm.

210. Kathleen Holton, "Actually, MSG Is Not Safe for Everyone (Op-Ed)," 2014, http://www.livescience.com/47931-msg-not-safe-for-everyone.html.

211. Battling the MSG Myth, "EmilyS MSG Recovery Story," 2009, http://www.msgmyth.com/discus/messages/1557/2057.html?1256917616.

212. American Heart Association, "FAQs of Atrial Fibrillation," https://www.heart.org/idc/groups/heart-public/@wcm/@hcm/documents/downloadable/ucm_424424.pdf.

213. Broadwith, Phillip, "Glutamate," Royal Society of Chemistry, June 2011, http://www.rsc.org/images/IC0411-glutamate-food_tcm18-233514.pdf.

214. Truth in Labeling, "History of invention and use of MSG," http://www.truthinlabeling.org/IVhistoryOfUse.html.

215. Blaylock, op. cit., p. 34.

216. Truth in Labeling, "History of invention and use of MSG," http://www.truthinlabeling.org/IVhistoryOfUse.html.

217. Adam Marcus, "MSG linked to weight gain," 2011, http://www.reuters.com/article/us-msg-linked-weight-gain-idUSTRE74Q5SJ20110527.

218. Makoto Fujimoto et al., "A Dietary Restriction Influences the Progression But Not the Initiation of MSG-Induced Nonalcoholic Steatohepatitis," *Journal of Medicinal Food*, March 2014, http://online.liebertpub.com/doi/abs/10.1089/jmf.2012.0029.

219. Blaylock, op. cit., p. 80.

220. Blaylock, p. 43.

221. Ibid, p. 14.

222. Simontacchi, Carol, *The Crazy Makers* (New York: Tarcher Putnam, 2000), p. 97.

223. Blaylock, op. cit., p. 35.

224. Ibid, p. 55.

225. Ibid, p. xix.

226. Simontacchi, op. cit., p. 96.

227. Blaylock, op. cit., pp. 37–38.

228. Ibid, pp. xvii, 170.

229. Linda Bonvie, "How the misrepresentation of a trusted product name could land you in the ER," 2014, http://foodidentitytheft.com/how-the-misrepresentation-of-a-trusted-product-name-could-land-you-in-the-er/.

PARTIALLY HYDROGENATED OILS

230. Sabrina Tavernise, "F.D.A. Sets 2018 Deadline to Rid Foods of Trans Fats," *New York Times*, June 2015, http://www.nytimes.com/2015/06/17/health/fda-gives-food-industry-three-years-eliminate-trans-fats.html.

231. Department of Health and Human Services Food and Drug Administration, "Final Determination Regarding Partially Hydrogenated Oils," https://s3.amazonaws.com/public-inspection.federalregister.gov/2015-14883.pdf.

232. Sarah McClelland et al., "Conjugated linoleic acid suppresses the migratory and inflammatory phenotype of the monocyte/macrophage cell," *Atherosclerosis*, July 2010, http://www.atherosclerosis-journal.com/article/S0021-9150(10)00101-2/abstract.

233. Ibid.

234. Ibid.

235. Sabrina Tavernise, "F.D.A. Sets 2018 Deadline to Rid Foods of Trans Fats," *New York Times*, June 2015, http://www.nytimes.com/2015/06/17/health/fda-gives-food-industry-three-years-eliminate-trans-fats.html?_r=0.

236. Todd Zwillich, "Panel Says No Amount of Trans Fat Is Safe," http://www.preventdisease.com/news/articles/no_transfat_safe.shtml.

237. Marisa Schultz, "FDA to spread Bloomberg's trans–fat ban nationwide," *New York Post*, June 2015, http://nypost.com/2015/06/01/fda-to-spread-bloombergs-trans-fat-ban-nationwide/.

238. Sabrina Tavernise, "F.D.A. Sets 2018 Deadline to Rid Foods of Trans Fats," *New York Post*, June 2015, http://www.nytimes.com/2015/06/17/health/fda-gives-food-industry-three-years-eliminate-trans-fats.html?_r=0.

239. Eliza Barclay, "When Zero Doesn't Mean Zero: Trans Fats Linger In Food," *NPR*, August 2014, http://www.npr.org/sections/thesalt/2014/08/28/343971652/trans-fats-linger-stubbornly-in-the-food-supply.

240. Sally Robertson, "Study warns that trans fats may be bad for the memory," 2014, http://www.news-medical.net/news/20141120/Study-warns-that-trans-fats-may-be-bad-for-the-memory.aspxC.

241. Linda Joyce Forristal, "The Rise and Fall of Crisco," http://www.motherlindas.com/crisco.htm.

242. Ibid.

243. Ethan Trex, "The Surprisingly Interesting History of Margarine," Mental Floss, 2010, http://mentalfloss.com/article/25638/surprisingly-interesting-history-margarine.

244. Stephan Guyenet, "Butter, Margarine and Heart Disease," 2008, http://wholehealthsource.blogspot.com/2008/12/butter-margarine-and-heart-disease.html.

245. Nina Teicholz, "The Questionable Link Between Saturated Fat and Heart Disease," *Wall Street Journal*, May 2014, http://www.wsj.com/articles/SB10001424052702303678404579533760760481486.

246. Stephan Guyenet, "Butter, Margarine and Heart Disease," 2008, http://wholehealthsource.blogspot.com/2008/12/butter-margarine-and-heart-disease.html.

247. Levenstein, Harvey, *Fear of Food: A History of Why We Worry About What We Eat* (Chicago: University of Chicago Press, 2012), p. 144.

248. Marian Burros, "Margarine Choices: A Guide for Consumers," *New York Times*, November 1984, http://www.nytimes.com/1984/11/21/garden/margarine-choices-a-guide-for-consumers.html?pagewanted=all.

249. Fleischmanns.com, "Our Spreads," http://www.fleischmanns.com/our-spreads.jsp.

250. Brady Dannis, "The 100-year-old scientist who pushed the FDA to ban artificial trans fat," *Washington Post*, June 2015, https://www.washingtonpost.com/news/to-your-health/wp/2015/06/16/the-100-year-old-scientist-who-pushed-the-fda-to-ban-artificial-trans-fat/.

251. Jack Bouboushian, "Researcher Wants FDA to Ban Trans Fat," *Courthouse News Service*, August 2013, http://www.courthousenews.com/2013/08/13/60216.htm.

252. Melissa Clark, "Once a Villain, Coconut Oil Charms the Health Food World," *New York Times*, March 2011, http://www.nytimes.com/2011/03/02/dining/02Appe.html?pagewanted=all.

253. I. A. Prior et al., "Cholesterol, coconuts, and diet on Polynesian atolls: a natural experiment: the Pukapuka and Tokelau island studies." *American Journal of Clinical Nutrition*, August 1981, http://ajcn.nutrition.org/content/34/8/1552.short.

254. Kris Gunnars, "10 Proven Health Benefits of Coconut Oil," https://authoritynutrition.com/top-10-evidence-based-health-benefits-of-coconut-oil/.

255. Sayer Ji, "MCT Fats Found In Coconut Oil Boost Brain Function In Only One Dose," Green Med Info, 2013, http://www.greenmedinfo.com/blog/mct-fats-found-coconut-oil-boost-brain-function-only-one-dose.

256. North Carolina Egg Association, "Good News For Eggs In 2015 Dietary Guidelines For Americans," http://ncegg.org/blog/good-news-eggs-2015-dietary-guidelines-americans/.

257. Mary Brophy Marcus, "Are full-fat dairy foods better for you after all?," CBS News, April 2016, http://www.cbsnews.com/news/full-fat-dairy-foods-diabetes-obesity-risk/.

258. Ibid.

rBGH or rBST

259. Robin, Marie-Monique, *The World According to Monsanto* (New York: The New Press, 2010), p. 91.

260. Ibid, p. 105.

261. Rick North and Martin Donohoe, "Open Letter to FDA: Why Monsanto's Genetically Engineered Bovine Growth Hormone Needs to Be Banned," 2007, https://www.organicconsumers.org/news/open-letter-fda-why-monsantos-genetically-engineered-bovine-growth-hormone-needs-be-banned.

262. Edward Group, "8 Shocking Facts about Bovine Growth Hormone," 2014, http://www.globalhealingcenter.com/natural-health/8-shocking-facts-bovine-growth-hormone/.

263. Ibid.

264. Robin, op. cit., pp. 97, 98.

265. Ibid, p. 90.

266. Innvista, "Milk," http://www.innvista.com/health/foods/genetically-engineered-foods/milk/.

267. Robyn O'Brien, "Dirty Dairy: Why Breyer's Ice Cream Dumped Artificial Growth Hormones," 2015, http://robynobrien.com/dirty-dairy-why-breyers-ice-cream-dumped-artificial-growth-hormones.

268. Mateusz Perkowski, "Dairymen reject rBST largely on economic grounds," *Capital Press*, December 2013, http://www.capitalpress.com/article/20131210/ARTICLE/131219995.

269. Robin, op. cit., pp. 109–110.

270. The Organic & Non-GMO Report, "Monsanto urges FDA to stop 'misleading' rBST-free labeling," May 2007, http://www.non-gmoreport.com/articles/may07/misleading_rBST-free_labeling.php.

271. Sylvia E. Simson, "Ohio Withdraws Dairy Labeling Regulation", 2011, http://product-liability.weil.com/food-and-beverage/ohio-withdraws-dairy-labeling-regulation/.

272. GRACE Communications Foundation Communications Foundation, "What is rBGH (and rBTS?)" http://www.sustainabletable.org/797/rbgh.

273. "Dairymen reject rBST…", op. cit.

274. USDA, Dairy Cattle Management Practices in the United States, 2014, https://www.aphis.usda.gov/animal_health/nahms/dairy/downloads/dairy14/Dairy14_dr_PartI.pdf.

275. Robin, op. cit., p. 114.

276. Ibid, p. 122.

277. GRACE Communications Foundation Communications Foundation, "What is rBGH (and rBTS?)" http://www.sustainabletable.org/797/rbgh.

INDEX